Arthritis in the knee, os
knee.

Knee arthritis types, k
stretches, treatments, home remedies, knee
replacements and knee braces all covered.

by

Robert Rymore

Published by IMB Publishing 2013

Disclaimer

Information in this book has been written by the author to serve a purpose of informing and educating the reader on knee arthritis. The author and/or publisher do not take any responsibility for the accuracy, precision and quality of the information contained herein. The author declares the use of any information contained in this book to be the reader's responsibility and call.

The websites, medications, service providers, books, and other mentioning of brand names in this book does not mean recommendation or endorsement by the author and/or publisher. Their mention is for sharing information with the reader pertaining to knee arthritis. Any repercussions occurring due to the use of these aforementioned is the reader's liability.

Any medication, treatment and suggestions used in this book are not intended for self-diagnosis and treatment. Consult your doctor for any medical enquiries and complaints. Failure to abide by the terms of use of this book and consequences resulting from this are the reader's accountability.

Furthermore, distribution and/or use of copyrighted information in this book without the author's permission is prosecutable by law.

Table of Contents

Preface

Robert Rymore is a researcher on medical subjects. He writes medical educational books in a relaxed, easy-to-understand way. This book on knee arthritis is one of his many, which are written for the sole purpose of educating the reader.

Having had knee arthritis hit one of his own has prompted Robert's writing of this particular book. His aunt Lucy is a 69-year-old lady, somewhat overweight. She developed osteoporosis early due to having had both her ovaries and uterus removed at the age of 40. For 3 years now, she suffers from severe osteoarthritis in both of her knees, and was unable to walk due to severe pain. She tried almost all available pain-relieving treatment modalities up until 4 months ago, when she had a total knee replacement on her right knee. Currently she is doing well, continuing with physiotherapy, pain relief treatment and is waiting for her specialist's go-ahead on surgery of the other knee.

Millions of people are struggling with knee arthritis. Robert's experience with a close family member has heightened his efforts to dig deep into many archives to research about knee arthritis. Any other individuals that may be in the same situation as Robert's aunt will benefit from this book.

This knee arthritis guide covers several types of knee arthritis. The development, symptoms, and treatment options for rheumatoid arthritis, osteoarthritis, gout arthritis, septic arthritis and post-traumatic arthritis, specifically for the knee are included. It is a very well researched and informative guide to anyone looking for answers on knee arthritis.

Foreword

My longtime colleague Robert has done justice to this book, as he always does to all his published books. After reading this book's draft, I can say that he covered everything that anyone looking for information on knee arthritis should know about. This particular book on knee arthritis is of personal interest to me; having an early form of arthritis in my left knee, I will surely try the tips and suggestions in this book. Great work, Robert, and thank you for coming through with this read at my exact time of need.

Susan Turner
Medical researcher
London, 2013

Acknowledgements

This book is dedicated to my aunt Lucy, who has been an inspiration of braveness and courage. My gratitude also extends to my proofreader, my typist and secretary, for their excellent work. Lastly, to my family, I glow because of your love and support.

Introduction

The Center for Disease Control and Prevention (CDC) in 2007-2009 has estimated arthritis to be the most common cause of disability. In their data sheet for the same period of time, approximately 49.9 million U.S. adults were reported to have been diagnosed by a doctor with having arthritis. This accounted for about 22.2 % of the population, and an estimated $128 billion in annual medical costs.

Also in the community are some people who have self-diagnosed arthritis, making the 22.2% prevalence a fraction of the possible actual statistics. The high costs of medical care, and the reduced productivity that results from the high rate of disability, is a great burden on the economy.

Arthritis affects mostly adults, from around 30 years of age and more, although young age groups can also be affected. Female gender has a 2-3 times risk for the development of arthritis in a lifetime, in comparison to the male gender. In general, arthritis can strike anyone at any time regardless of their age, ethnicity, stamina and geographical location. Some risk factors, however, may alter the prevalence of this medical condition. Obesity is one of the risk factors of arthritis development, which occurs at double the rate in an obese individual when compared to those who are of normal weight.

Different kinds of arthritis exist, differentiated by their pathological development and location. Rheumatoid arthritis, osteoarthritis, gout arthritis, post-traumatic arthritis and septic arthritis are the kinds that are going to be discussed in this book, specified to the knee joint.

In a 2013 report, the Arthritis Research UK Primary Care Centre has analyzed the data of people who consulted about osteoarthritis in general practice over a period of 7 years. It is estimated that approximately 8.75 million people in the U.K. sought treatment for osteoarthritis. The impact of arthritis is so grave that the Arthritis Society has estimated more Canadians to have died from arthritis than from HIV/AIDS, asthma and melanoma. Arthritis symptoms include pain, difficulties in walking and working, with general body illness causing disability.

The knee and the hip are the most affected joints of the human body. This is partly because these joints are the main weight bearers of the body and are responsible for coordination and locomotion. From the 2013 report of the Arthritis Research UK Primary Care Centre, the knee was affected in approximately 18% of the population who sought treatment of osteoarthritis, compared to 8% for the hip, which was the second highest.

In this guide knee arthritis is deeply described in a laid back fashion, which allows effortless interpretation by the user. For better clarity, the knee as a structure is first discussed, along with its anatomical makeup and function. It also explains the exact differences between a normal knee and an arthritic one. Further on, it reviews the different kinds of knee arthritis, explaining pain relief measures for each and their available treatment modalities. This book is bursting with tips and suggestions on knee arthritis, especially home remedies and some advice on how to improve function through exercise, when one suffers from knee arthritis. It is a joy to announce that besides the 5 main knee arthritis to be discussed in this book, 2 additional forms of arthritis - namely reactive arthritis and psoriatic arthritis - have been added on request. Brace yourself for a thorough insight on knee arthritis.

Chapter 1) The knee as a structure

1) Anatomy of the knee

When we squat, the knee joint supports 6-8 times our body weight. The knee joint is the largest joint in the body, and it is used in all activities that require movement from one point to another, e.g. walking and jogging. Looking at its functions, and the amount of weight that it is required to support, the knee joint is therefore one of the most vulnerable joints in the body.

Its anatomical makeup is not only articulating bones, but it is a complicated construct held together by an extensive network of ligaments and muscles. Blood vessels and nerves are located at the back of the knee, where to some extent they are vulnerable to injury if the knee joint is to be injured. The knee joint is a synovial joint. This means that it is lined by a synovial membrane that produces synovial fluid for joint lubrication. The knee can also be called a modified hinge joint, as it allows movement of only bending and straightening with a slight sideways rotation. The knee joint consists of 2 joints, the tibiofemoral joint and the patellofemoral joint. The tibiofemoral joint is an articulation between the thigh bone and the shin bone, whereas the patellofemoral joint exists between the thigh bone and the kneecap. The kneecap is located in a groove between the 2 distal bulges of the thigh bone; the femoral condyles.

Some books state that 4 bones form the knee joint: the thigh bone (femur), shin bone (tibia), kneecap (patella), and the outer shin bone (fibula). The fibula, however, does not really participate in the knee articulation, but still supports the joint construct. There are therefore 3 articulating bones . On the surface of these articulating bones is a white, smooth and shiny surface called cartilage. Cartilage is very important for the knee joint mobility to be friction-free, thus also pain-free.

The knee is part of what is called an appendicular skeleton, where together with the pelvis, hip, leg, ankle and foot, they form the lower limb. The lower limb is, in turn, the unit used in locomotion.

The knee joint, in detail, is made up of bones, ligaments, tendons, cartilage, joint capsule, and the neurovascular bundle.

a) The bones of the knee

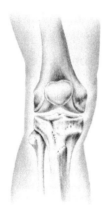

Bones are made up of collagen, which is a protein substance abundant in all tissues of the body. Collagen, together with other substances in the matrix, forms bone. There are 2 types of bone, compact bone and spongy bone. Compact bone consists of a hard, outer surface with a spongy, bony marrow cavity. Spongy bone is soft and porous, to allow for movement of fluids within it, e.g. blood in the bone marrow. The bones that form the knee are compact, long bones:

A) Femur - the largest, longest and strongest bone in the body. It is also known as the thigh bone. It consists of a head, which is located at the hip, a shaft and condyles. Femoral condyles are the 2 large knobs located at the lower end of the femur bone. These condyles articulate with the kneecap to form the patellofemoral joint.

B) Tibia - found between the knee and the ankle, commonly known as the shin bone. The tibia is the second longest bone in the body, consisting of a smooth surface that articulates at the knee joint, which is called the tibial plateau. In the centre of this articulating surface is a spiky protuberance known as the tibial tubercle. This tibial tubercle divides the tibial plateau into medial and lateral plateaus. Medial means closer to the midline, as in the inside of the knee, whereas lateral means the outer surface. Just below the tibial plateau in the front is a protuberance called the tibial tuberosity. It is at this tuberosity where the patella tendon attaches, as it runs from its originating point at the kneecap. The tibia has a shaft in the middle and, at the distal end participates in formation of the ankle joint.

C) Fibula - a thin, long bone which runs parallel to the tibia. It is located on the lateral side of the leg. The fibula on its proximal part has a head - this fibular head articulates with the tibia. Though the fibula does not participate in the formation of the knee joint, its articulation with the tibia provides support to the knee joint. In its shape, the fibula also has a shaft in the middle, and its bottom end participates in the formation of the ankle joint.

D) Patella - not a long bone, and commonly known as the kneecap. It is a flat, triangular shaped sesamoid bone. The quadriceps muscle tendon attaches to the upper pole of the patella, and the patellar tendon at its lower pole. When the knee straightens and bends, the patella moves to relieve friction between the knee bones and muscles. The patella glides on the femoral condyles during this movement.

b) Knee tendons

Tendons are thick, fibrous tissues that are intermediates connecting muscles to bone. When muscles contract, the force they exert on the tendon is transferred to bones, hence facilitating locomotion. At the knee joint, there are 2 main tendons: the quadriceps and patellar. The 2 tendons form what is known as the extensor mechanism of the knee. The extensor mechanism of the knee basically means a way in which the knee straightens. The quadriceps tendon connects the quadriceps muscle to the kneecap. This attachment also helps to stabilize the kneecap in the femoral condyler groove, hence preventing its dislocation. The patellar tendon connects the kneecap to the shin bone, allowing the quadriceps muscle contraction forces to be further transferred to the shin, thus allowing the straightening of the leg. The patellar tendon is a ligament, since ligaments are collagen fibres connecting bone to bone.

c) Ligaments of the knee

The knee is a strong joint. Its stability owes greatly to the presence of its ligaments. A ligament is a fibrous collagen band that connects bone to bone. For optimal knee stability, different positions on the knee have different ligaments. Unlike tendons, which are flexible and a bit stretchy, ligaments are somewhat rigid and can snap if they are overstretched.

- **Medial collateral ligament (MCL)** - also known as the tibial collateral ligament, is a fibrous band that runs between the inner femur surface and the tibia. It helps resist stresses, and/or forces acting on the outer knee surface, which are called valgus forces.

- **Lateral collateral ligament (LCL)** - also called the fibular collateral ligament, is a ligament located on the outer surface of the knee, traveling from the lateral surface of the femur to the head of the fibula. It helps to stabilize the knee against inner surface stresses, which are called varus forces.

- **Posterior cruciate ligament (PCL)** - this ligament wraps around the anterior cruciate ligament, as it travels from the posterior tibial surface to the anterior of the femur. It prevents the backward gliding of the knee joint.

- **Anterior cruciate ligament (ACL)** – this ligament is very important as its injury may require an aggressive approach of surgery and rehabilitation. It is positioned from the front of the tibia to the back of the femur. It prevents the tibia from overextending to the front.

The cruciate ligaments have this name because they criss-cross in the middle of the knee joint.

d) Smooth running of the knee joint

The articulating bones of the knee joint are covered by articular cartilage. Articular cartilage is a white, shiny and smooth fibrous connective tissue. It protects the bones of a joint as they move. Besides cartilage, in the knee joint, on the tibial plateau is a C-shaped meniscus. A meniscus is made from a rubber-like material, which acts as a shock absorber. Like how the tibial plateau is divided into 2, the meniscus is also divided into the medial and lateral menisci. Menisci distribute weight over the whole surface of the tibial plateau, so that there is no weight overload.

The knee joint capsule is lined by a special membrane called synovium. This synovial membrane produces synovial fluid, which is an egg white–like, slippery substance that functions as a lubricant to the joint. The synovial fluid enhances the slipperiness of articular cartilage, estimated to be about 3 times more slippery if compared to skating on ice.

Other components such as bursae and plicae also contribute to joint smoothness. A bursa is a small, fluid-filled sac, which is found between muscles, tendons, ligaments and bone. Bursae cushion the knee joint. Approximately 13 bursae are found around the knee. The pre-patellar bursa is one of the main bursae of the knee. It is located in front of the knee, just under the skin. It protects the kneecap, and if injured can cause a painful condition known as bursitis. Besides bursae, plicae and fat pads also help to maintain the knee joint running smoothly. Plicae are synovial membrane folds.

e) Muscles around the knee

The knee function to bend and straighten is controlled by 2 muscle groups. These muscle groups are antagonistic; the flexor muscles bend the knee, while the extensor muscle group straightens the knee. The flexors, quadriceps muscle, consist of 4 muscles that join to form a common tendon; quadriceps tendon. They are located on the front of the thigh. They are called vastus lateralis, vastus medialis, vastus intermedialis and rectus femoris. The knee extensor muscle group, the hamstrings, is a group of 3 muscles known as semitendinosus, semimembranosus and biceps femoris. Overuse of these muscles can cause tendinitis, which is another source of pain around the knee.

f) The joint capsule

The joint capsule of the knee is continuous with the ligaments and encompasses the whole joint. It is a ligamentous, thick connective tissue, which is lined by synovium. Synovium provides nutrition to all the surrounding structures of the knee joint.

2) Knee pain

Knee pain is a common complaint by patients who visit the doctor's office. It affects all ages, but its occurrence can be influenced by certain risk factors. Risk factors to knee pain include sporting activities, aging, trauma and obesity.

Knee pain can be acute and/or may occur gradually over time. Torn ligaments, ruptured tendons, bone fractures and joint infection may result in pain that starts suddenly. Overuse injuries, e.g. tendonitis, bursitis and arthritis, take a more gradual, chronic picture of knee pain. Acute is defined as a condition occurring for 3 weeks or less, whereas chronic is beyond 3 weeks, which could be months or years. Many types of minor knee pain respond well to self-care measures. Physical therapy, exercises and knee braces are amongst the things that can relieve knee pain. In severe cases, however, surgical repair may be required.

3) Differentiating knee pain

Differentiating knee pain means pinpointing the number one cause of any knee pain. This is not an easy task as many reasons exist as to why one might feel knee pain. Differential diagnosis, abbreviated as ddx, is done by doctors and requires complete history taking, a thorough physical examination, and a wide range of medical tests. Differentiating knee pain is important to rule out any immediate medical conditions, which require an aggressive approach to treatment, e.g. a septic arthritis in children and immune-suppressed adults. Some of the common causes of knee pain are listed below.

- Knee ligament injury

Any one of the 2 collateral ligaments and/or cruciates can be injured by trauma. This trauma can be a result of a fall, a road accident, skating or skiing accidents and other sporting activities. Ligament injuries cause a sudden onset of pain, and are noticed immediately as soon as they occur. Most often, the knee ligaments are torn when an overstretch is applied in any direction on a fixed knee.

An MCL injury gives pain and localized tenderness on the inside of the knee. An LCL injury results in a sharp pain and tenderness on the outer surface of the knee joint. Any cruciate ligament injury causes pain that is located deep within the knee joint. A snapping sound may be reported by the patient. It is felt at the time of a ligament tearing. Swelling and warmth of the knee may also be noted. At a particular time, one or more ligaments may be injured.

Knee ligament injury can be graded as mild, moderate, and severe. Mild means a few fibres of the ligament are torn; however, the other ligament fibres are still intact, which is called a minor sprain. A moderate ligament sprain has a few more fibres torn, but otherwise, some are also still intact. A severe ligament injury will result in the complete tearing of the ligament. Giving way when walking is an indicative sign of knee ligament instability, hence injury. For instance, if the PCL is injured, a patient will feel like the shin bone is overextending backwards when he/she walks, which is called hyperextension.

The RICE method is one of the treatment plans that is initiated when a ligament is injured. Rest, Ice, Compression and Elevation significantly reduces pain and promotes healing. Resting is of importance, hence crutches may be required for a few weeks.

Analgesics, usually non-steroidal anti-inflammatory drugs, are prescribed to help ease the swelling and pain. However, surgical repair may be necessary. Surgical approaches involve the suturing of the torn ligaments, grafting and/or their reconstruction.

- Torn meniscus

The meniscus can be torn with shearing stress of rotation applied on a fixed knee in rapid motion. Meniscal tear is a very common sports injury. A patient may complain of popping and catching of the torn meniscus upon moving the joint. Its onset is sudden, with occasional knee swelling and warmth. A doctor can perform diagnosis-supporting tests, e.g. the grinding test. Other medical tests are required to substantiate the diagnosis, where routing X-rays, arthroscopy and MRI can be of benefit.

- Fractures and dislocations

Any one of the 3 articulating bones that form the knee joint can be broken by trauma. Road traffic accidents, sporting activities and falls all contribute to high energy, which can result in fractures and/or dislocations around the knee joint. Fractures around the knee often require surgical treatment so as to maintain the joint congruency, without which early arthritis can appear, which is known as post-traumatic arthritis.

Also around the knee, it is possible for one to dislocate the kneecap, or the femur over the tibia. This dislocation can be complete, or partial, which is called a sublaxation. Knee joint sublaxation or dislocation is an emergency, which requires urgent orthopedic reduction. Dislocations often result in injury to the nerves and blood vessels, as these structures pass in close proximity to the femur and tibia at the back of the knee joint. Early reduction of the joint is therefore necessary to prevent stretching of this neurovascular bundle. X-rays are usually adequate to diagnose fractures and dislocations. However, other tests such as angiography and MRI may be required in case of a simultaneous neurovascular bundle injury.

- Bursitis

When a bursa becomes inflamed, a condition known as bursitis results. Bursitis causes pain, swelling and tenderness over the location of the bursa, e.g. pre-patellar bursa in front of the knee. Bursitis at the knee is common in individuals who kneel a lot, thus its other name is "housemaid's knee." Kneeling on the floor or carpet causes friction and rubbing of the skin and the bursa underneath it. Clinical examination and patient history are adequate to make a diagnosis. Analgesics, ice packs and local cortisone injections are useful in relieving pain.

- Tendonitis

Overuse injuries of the tendons of the knee can result in tendonitis, which is inflammation of the tendons. Patellar tendonitis, which is also known as the "jumper's knee," is often encountered in individuals who play sports that involve jumping, e.g. basketball and volleyball. The knee can become swollen, warm and tender, though the most tender spot is just over the affected tendon. Quadriceps tendonitis and hamstring tendonitis are amongst the other tendonitis types that occur around the knee. Implementing the RICE method, physiotherapy and other pain treatment options available for tendonitis can be done. These treatment options include corticosteroid injections, glucose injections, Botox injections, ultrasound and shockwave therapy. Massage and daily stretches are among the leading home remedies performed by most sufferers to relieve pain. A complete patient history, thorough physical examination and special tests can accurately diagnose this condition. However, other additional medical investigations may be necessary for differential diagnosis. These include routine X-rays, blood work and at times an MRI.

- Baker's cyst

A Baker's cyst, or popliteal cyst, is a swelling that protrudes at the back of the knee. It is a protrusion of the synovial membrane, and hence it is fluid-filled. Popliteal cysts are common and may result from any condition that can cause knee swelling, e.g. arthritis, cartilage tear and other knee problems. A Baker's cyst may get complicated by rupturing and oozing fluid into the muscles at the back of the leg. Very often joint aspiration, corticosteroid injections and surgical removal suffice for its complete resolution.

- Chondromalacia patella

Chondromalacia patella is often called the patellofemoral syndrome. From the previous text, our understanding is that the patellofemoral joint is formed by the patella, and the femur. Both surfaces of these 2 bones are covered by articular cartilage. In chondromalacia patella, the articulating cartilage on the underside of the patella is abnormally soft, causing pain at the front of the knee. The patellofemoral syndrome is among the leading causes of chronic knee pain. Also, in chondromalacia patella, the patella is pulled to the side during knee straightening; normally it should be tracking straight on the patellar groove of the femur. This sideway position of the patella in the patellofemoral syndrome causes constant irritation, inflammation and pain. Risk factors of this condition include being female, having a short patella, and predisposing cartilage disorders. Symptoms are often pain, which is felt during knee joint movement, a strange feeling of 'tightness' in the knee joint, and reduced quadriceps muscle strength. X-rays and MRIs can substantiate the cartilage tear behind the patella and therefore aid in diagnosing this condition. Treatment involves strengthening the quadriceps muscles to help the patella to track on the femoral patella groove as it should. Some sufferers improve with a cortisone shot, otherwise physiotherapy is the mainstay of its treatment.

- Others

There are still many more conditions that require differentiating in knee pain. Blood in the knee joint (haemarthrosis) is one of them, which occurs after trauma, or spontaneously in patients with blood clotting disorders like haemophilia, and/or those on blood thinners like aspirin and warfarin. Connective tissue disorders may also result in knee joint pain; systemic lupus erythematosus is one such disorder. Cartilage tears, Osgood-Schlatter disease, tumors and referred pain from the hip or foot are other reasons as to why knee pain may occur. The leading cause of knee pain, however, is knee arthritis. This book is centered on this particular cause of knee pain.

4) Medical tests for knee pain

In the doctor's office, a complete history taking and a thorough physical examination are done. These should provide the most probable cause of the knee pain, which is called a provisional diagnosis. Medical investigations are carried out to confirm the provisional diagnosis, and to differentiate any other candidate conditions.

- History

History of a disease means all events that occurred up to the development of the symptoms of knee pain. In the history of knee pain, there is often a report of an injury, whether a fall, an accident or a sports-associated injury. Complaints of swelling, warmth and tenderness are the most prevalent in sufferers of knee pain. However, most chronic and gradual causes of knee pain like arthritis lack a history of trauma. Other concomitant diseases may be noted, such as diabetes mellitus, hypertension and lupus. Previous diseases may also result in what is known as reactive arthritis, even after their complete resolution. This is true for streptococcal B infections, especially tonsillitis. Medications that a patient has been taking and/or is still being taken should be reported. Previous knee surgeries and indications that led to the surgery should be discussed. If there are any investigations that were done, their results should be produced, together with information of the attending doctor. All of these points are relevant for a physician to realize the extent of your complaints and all possible candidate diseases to your knee pain.

- Physical examination

During physical examination, a physician does special tests to evaluate the extent of your knee pain. All the previously discussed components of the knee are checked. The ligaments, in a varus and valgus stress test, and function of the knee are checked by testing the free range of motion. Any meniscal tear is confirmed by the grinding test (also known as McMurray's test), and crepitations on moving the patella or the knee joint are noted. All muscles are tested for strength and function. Sensation of the skin overlying the knee is also evaluated. This is important because peripheral neurological disorders also contribute to knee pain and knee arthritis development. If the knee joint is swollen, joint aspiration may be done to check for the contents of the effusion, which could be blood, synovial fluid, pus and their combinations. This procedure, however, should be done under sterile conditions; otherwise infective agents may be introduced into the joint. Checking of the position of the knees when walking is necessary, as conditions like knock-knee or bowlegs predispose the joint to arthritis. After a complete physical examination, a physician should come up with the leading disease condition that causes your knee pain.

- Investigations

An MRI, if readily available, will show most joint tissue injuries, e.g. isolated ligament injuries, bone infarction, vascular injury and cartilage tears to mention just a few. A downside to an MRI is that it's an expensive test. If MRI cannot be accessed, a plain X-ray in different views should be done. A lateral view excludes osteoarthritis, loose bodies and tumors, while other views like a weight-bearing X-ray and an antero-posterior (AP) view may show joint effusion, osteophytes, joint space changes and cartilage defects. At times, soon after injury, especially in acute conditions, a plain X-ray film may not reveal the pathology. Repeating the X-ray after 2 weeks is recommended in such cases. An ultrasound scan is good in cases of joint effusion, especially in young age groups, although ultrasound scans are rarely ordered, as almost always a radiologist will suggest another investigation like MRI as an end note.

Blood tests are important, but these blood works are specific. For instance, uric acid is often checked in gout arthritis; inflammatory markers like rheumatoid factor in rheumatoid arthritis. Other non-specific blood works include a full blood count (FBC), erythrocyte sedimentation rate (ESR), and C-reactive protein (CRP). These are usually elevated in acute knee infections, e.g. septic arthritis and/or tumors. However, these markers may be normal in chronic knee diseases.

Still, on additional blood tests, some other forms of arthritis like reactive arthritis, which is part of the seronegative spondyloarthropathies may require human leukocytic antigen gene (HLA-B27) to be checked, though its presence is not confirmatory for the disease. However, HLA-B27 may be used as a predictor of a severe form of reactive arthritis.

Depending on the primary foci of infection, which led to the development of other arthritis types, e.g. reactive arthritis, urinalysis may be ordered for urinary tract infections, stool analysis for gastrointestinal diseases, and sputum for respiratory tract conditions. A referral to the urologist, ophthalmologist, or a genitourinary specialist may be required for a diagnosis to be reached *(see additional arthritis section).*

Aspirate from a joint is worth doing, but it should not be performed in a joint with prosthesis, if the knee has not any effusion, and when the overlying skin has an infection. Joint aspirate can be tested for crystals in gout and pseudo-gout of the knee, microbial agents in case of an infection, together with the response to specific antibiotics. Knee arthroscopy is yet another investigation that can be performed as a diagnostic test and/or for treatment. Arthroscopy allows for keyhole surgical intervention to knee conditions. On diagnosis, arthritis, meniscal injury, ligament injury and cartilage defects can be seen clearly. A CT scan is a good diagnostic tool in conditions that involve the bone, e.g. fractures, a loose body in the joint, or a tumor. Where tumors are diagnosed, a TC99 bone scan of the whole body is an excellent addition. This test will help localize other zones with a tumor or metastasis.

Chapter 2) Knee arthritis

1) What is knee arthritis?

A model of knee arthritis:

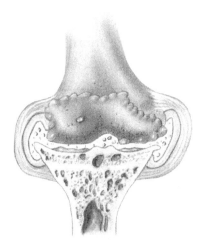

Knee arthritis is the inflammation and wearing off of the knee joint. This inflammation can affect 1 or both joints, and has no specific age for its development. The main sign of knee arthritis is knee pain, which is called arthralgia. There are estimated to be as many as 100 different identified types of arthritis. Many other kinds are still being discovered. The causes of knee arthritis are specific to each type of arthritis. This means that the way in which the knee joint wears and tears in arthritis is different in different forms of arthritis. To understand the causes of arthritis, one has to learn the pathophysiological mechanisms of development of the arthritis in question. Autoimmune origins result in rheumatoid arthritis and SLE (systemic lupus erythematosus), whereas abnormalities in protein metabolism result in gout or pseudo gout. Hereditary influences may play a role directly or indirectly and to some extent may cause osteoarthritis. A few years after knee trauma, an individual may be predisposed to post-traumatic arthritis. Infections of the knee joint can affect any individual, but their risk of occurrence is greater in immune compromised individuals, e.g. individuals on long-term corticosteroid treatment.

Therefore, each knee arthritis type has a specific pathogenesis, features, progression, treatment and complications. This book aims to describe and explain 5 main types of knee arthritis, namely osteoarthritis, rheumatoid arthritis, gout arthritis, post-traumatic arthritis and septic arthritis.

2) Knee arthritis epidemiology

In the United States, 28% of 45+ year-olds suffer from knee arthritis. In a certain Russian study, about 12,7% of children from a group of 5.490 children suffer from arthralgia. In Canada, according to the Arthritis Facts and Statistics by the Arthritis Society, about 4,5 million people aged 15 years and older have been reported to have arthritis. Obesity increases the chance of knee arthritis development, and it also heightens its progression. Postmenopausal women are affected more, due to osteoporosis being dominant in this group of individuals. Of all these reported knee arthritis, osteoarthritis is the leading type. Osteoarthritis accounts for a greater percent of all knee replacements in Canada.

An early detection of arthritis will allow early intervention of measures that slow down its progression. Sadly, there is no cure for knee arthritis, but vast methods of symptom relief are available. Even with symptomatic relief, knee arthritis progression is still a common cause of disability.

3) Types of knee arthritis

In the U.S., 67 million people are estimated to be suffering from arthritis by the year 2030. People long ago used to think that arthritis symptoms result from the same cause, hence they were initiating treatment plans that were the same in all types of arthritis. The discovery of more than 100 arthritis types automatically cancelled that notion, necessitating a specific treatment plan for each individual arthritis type. Each type calls for a different treatment regimen. This means that correct diagnosis is the key to an effective treatment.

Besides the usual known rheumatoid arthritis, osteoarthritis and septic arthritis, other rare kinds of arthritis include: psoriatic arthritis, reactive arthritis, lupus, idiopathic juvenile arthritis, and haemorrhagic arthritis.

Lupus arthritis is a frequent manifestation of systemic lupus erythematosus (SLE). SLE is an autoimmune disease in which the antibodies and complement system of an individual's immunity attacks tissues of the body. Juvenile arthritis affects children, and at times the reasons for its occurrence are unknown, hence the term "idiopathic." Haemorrhagic arthritis occurs when blood enters the joints, causing irritation and arthritic inflammatory changes. Hemophilia and sickle cell disease are conditions that often cause blood to accumulate in joints, resulting in pain, tenderness and swelling. Psoriasis is a scaly, red and white patched skin condition that also manifests as joint pain, what is called psoriatic arthritis. The skin lesions that often affect the knees and elbows precede the arthritis in the majority of cases, though it can also occur vice versa.

The understanding of a specific kind of arthritis that is affecting a sufferer is of importance if one is to benefit from treatment. The next chapter discusses in detail some knee arthritis types.

Chapter 3) Knee arthritis types in detail

1) Osteoarthritis of the knee

Osteoarthritis (OA) is the leading form of knee arthritis. In some other books it is known as degenerative arthritis of the knee. It is a slowly progressing, degenerative condition that affects the whole knee. OA usually affects large joints of the body, where the knee is its main target followed by the hip. 85% of all knee prosthesis surgeries are carried out because of OA.

The occurrence of OA increases with age, where 6% of adults at the age of 30 have radiologic features of OA. 27 million Americans are estimated to have OA, and more than 60% of these sufferers are women.

a) So what is OA?

In a normal joint, there are mechanisms that allow smooth mobility within the joint; these have been described in the previous chapter. In OA, one component, cartilage, is damaged, eroded and no longer provides a smooth glide within the joint during movement. Due to this, the bones of the knee joint rub against one another. This rubbing creates more erosions and wearing off of the articular cartilage, resulting in pain. In an attempt to repair the injury, new bone forms on the margins of the bones of the knee, forming bony spurs and osteophytes. These osteophytes can break off and move freely in the joint as free bodies, causing more joint irritation and pain.

b) What causes knee OA?

Aging is the most common cause, although one misconception is that knee OA is a disease of the elderly. Almost everyone in their lifetime eventually develops OA of some degree, since collagen within the joint tissues degenerates with time. However, some factors do increase the possibilities of knee OA development. These include the following:

Age - as a person gets older, the collagen components of cartilage lose some cells, and hence a few chondrocytes remain. These chondrocytes do not have the ability to divide by mitosis. This characteristic of cartilage affects its healing ability as one gets older. Lack of healing means lack of repair after any injury.

Weight - knees hold about 8 times your body weight. Being obese increases this weight significantly. It is said that every pound you gain increases weight load on the knees by 4 pounds.

Gender - postmenopausal women have a greater risk of developing knee OA.

Heredity - inborn abnormalities in the alignment of the lower limbs and knees can predispose an individual to knee OA. Every individual has a weight-bearing angle, if the body is viewed in an upright position. Any deviations of this angle from the norm may result in knee OA.

RSIs - repetitive stress injuries occur in individuals who do certain sporting activities that require overuse of the knee joints, e.g. weightlifting. The same applies to people with jobs that require them to be repeating the same motion with their knees, e.g. kneeling or squatting. This overuse keeps the knees in a constant strain and does not allow for rest. A fatigued joint will soon lose internal balance and sustain injury.

Concomitant diseases - metabolic conditions like diabetes mellitus, endocrine disorders, and people with rheumatism have a greater chance of developing OA.

Injury - individuals who sustain major knee trauma develop knee OA over a period of 10 years. Thus, if an individual has an injury at the age of 13, knee OA will develop as early as 23 years of age.

Peripheral neuropathy - may result in arthritis, especially where loss of sensation to the knee is reported. Pain is a protective mechanism of the body to injury. In cases of loss of sensation after nerve injury, one does not feel the joint pain that appears in early arthritis. The defensive behavior that is initiated by pain will be absent in such individuals, resulting in severe joint injury and deformation, which is known as a Charcot joint.

c) Signs and symptoms of OA of the knee

Knee arthralgia is the main complaint of most sufferers. This pain is usually felt in both knees, in and around the joint, increasing with activity, although may also be present even at rest. Night pain is indicative of an advanced stage of knee OA.

Knee swelling - due to repetitive irritation within the knee joint, a chronic inflammation is always present. This inflammation causes the synovial membrane to hypertrophy; besides, bony spurs and osteophytes increase the bulk, and give the knee a deformed appearance.

Joint stiffness and crackling sounds are another sign. Stiffness is often experienced in the morning, and when one sits for long periods of time.

Reduced range of motion (ROM) - due to pain, most sufferers avoid moving the affected knee joint. This causes muscles and tendons to contract, lose their elasticity, and in severe cases to contract into a fixed position.

Catching and locking of the knee during movement.

Tenderness - around the joint.

Muscle weakness and atrophy.

Finger changes - the last joints of the fingers (distal interphalangeal joints) may have swellings which are known as Heberden's nodes, while the proximal interphalangeal joints have Bouchard's nodes.

d) Diagnosis of knee OA

Medical history and physical examination can bring about the diagnosis of knee OA. However, medical tests are required to support this diagnosis, and to rule out any other disease conditions. X-rays are often adequate, as the narrowing of the joint space, subchondral cysts, subarticular sclerosis, bony spurs and osteophyte are positive findings. An MRI may be necessary, though not always. In cases of a huge knee effusion, joint aspiration (tapping) can be done. The aspirate is removed to relieve pain and for diagnostic purposes. Aspirate in cases of knee OA has no inflammatory cells, is clear and viscous. Blood works, the likes of FBC, ESR and CRP, are usually done as a routine. Liver function test (LFT) is required before starting NSAIDs (non-steroidal anti-inflammatory drugs)

e) Differential diagnosis

Referred pain from the hips or the lower back, bursitis, and other types of knee arthritis, e.g. septic arthritis, reactive arthritis such as Reiter's syndrome and viral arthritis, are other conditions that may present in knee OA.

f) Treatment of OA of the knee

There is no cure for knee OA, however, certain measures can be taken to relieve symptoms and prevent further knee damage.

The RICE method is initiated, even before confirmation of the knee OA diagnosis. 'R-Rest' avoids use of the knee in ways that elicit pain. 'I-Ice', applied on the knee in the form of ice packs for 20-30 minutes, many times a day, helps to reduce pain. Ice packs should always be wrapped in a cloth or towel, before applying them in contact with skin. If ice packs are applied directly on the skin, one might suffer from a thermal burn. Substitutes to ice packs are available on the market and include the Arctic Ease cryotherapy wrap found on Amazon.com. An Arctic Ease cryotherapy wrap will allow you to ice while on the move, eliminating the boredom of having to sit and ice.

'C-Compression', can be achieved by wearing a knee support or by using a knee brace. These have been shown to relieve pain since they temporarily prevent the joint from moving. 'E-Elevation', helps reduce swelling of the lower limb and the joint.

When the RICE method is being implemented, rest does not mean that one is completely immobile. Light stretches and exercises are a must to maintain knee joint function and full range of motion (FROM).

Over-the-counter pain medications like naproxen, Tylenol and ibuprofen can be bought from any pharmacy and/or shop. Additionally, dietary supplements like chondroitin sulphate and glucosamine have been shown in several studies to help relieve pain and improve joint function. Other options to pain treatment include corticosteroid shots and/or anesthetic agents, although often they are given as a combination. Studies have shown that repetitive cortisone injections may cause cartilage lysis (chondrolysis), therefore their use is limited to only 3 times per joint in a lifetime, given over several weeks and months. Hyaluronic acid injections are yet another option. Hyaluronic acid exists naturally in our joints. Injecting it into the joint is like replenishing the lost hyaluronic acid. This injection has been reported by some individuals to relieve pain for longer periods of time; 6 months to a year. The downside is that hyaluronic injections are expensive, and yet not everyone gets the anticipated relief.

The holistic approach to knee OA would evaluate the patient's function, occupation, mood, interactions in society, activities that one does in their spare time, and quality of life. A doctor may ask you what your concerns are about the diagnosis, your expectations from treatment, and a general test of your knowledge on knee OA. Anxiety and depression signs are also screened for, since their simultaneous occurrence with knee OA may determine the effort that an individual may have to put in to thrive. Also of importance is checking how the sufferer perceives pain, i.e. individual threshold/sensitivity to pain, and if the prescribed medications are giving any relief. Evaluation of what a patient thinks about the effects that knee OA has on their daily life, e.g. house chores, hobbies and sleep, are good markers of the extent of disability in an individual. Limitations to living are increased if one cannot perform daily individual chores like brushing teeth and buttoning a shirt.

Patient safety assessment requires the physician to clear the patient from any risks of further injury, e.g. a possibility of falling. Measures of reducing the risks should be applied if one is found to be within high risk parameters. A patient's beliefs and culture do influence the acceptance of particular treatment options. These too should be checked beforehand as they might assist the doctor to offer an individual treatment plan that will be effective on an individual basis. The perception of exercise and the understanding of why exercises are of importance in treatment of knee OA are to be explored. Adherence tests to exercise regimes should be performed and patients monitored to confirm that they are truly following through with the required steps, and that they are performing the exercises correctly. If other disease states are present, their treatment should also be optimal so as to relieve the body of all kinds of stress. Alternative treatments can also be added as combinations to other methods, or used separately. These include dietary manipulations like the use of flaxseeds and flax oil, acupuncture and physiotherapy. Different physiotherapy routines are to be discussed separately under the physiotherapy topic.

One point to be noted is that knee OA is not an emergency, so a physician owes it to the patient to give them an opportunity to make decisions after they have been thoroughly informed.

Conservative treatment options for knee OA are directed mainly at relieving pain and improving joint mobility and function. However, in situations where knee OA is in its advanced stages, surgery may be the only effective option.

Surgeries that can be performed for knee OA treatment include a wide variety, and the choice for their use depends on the indications of surgery. Knee surgery can be of 2 types, an open surgery or arthroscopic. Arthroscopy involves the use of a fiber optic gadget, which allows visualization of the inside of the joint and its manipulation. Removal of debris from the joint during a knee joint debridement, repairing of cartilage, meniscus and ligaments can be performed through a 1 cm keyhole. In situations where the patient has some misalignment of the lower limb, corrective osteotomies can be performed. An osteotomy for the knee joint can be done in 2 locations, on the proximal shin bone or the distal thigh bone.

For some individuals, cartilage grafts can be attempted, especially in the young age groups, though the effectiveness of this method requires more research. Knee arthroplasty is an option that has shown a good success rate. A surgeon removes the arthritic knee joint components and replaces them with artificial ones. These artificial components can be done partially, which means a single side is replaced, or totally, which means the whole joint is replaced by artificial elements. The material of the artificial implants can be plastic or metal - either way, there are many success stories. Recovery after a knee arthroplasty may take long, but it does put an end to the pain.

Total knee replacement prosthesis:

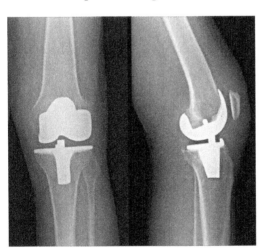

In situations where the joint does not allow for prosthesis, the knee joint may be fused in a procedure known as arthrodesis. Arthrodesis is a type of surgery done with the main aim of relieving pain. The articular cartilage of the bones of the knee is removed, and the thigh bone is then joined to the shin bone to form a continuous long bone after it heals. In other words, the joined site will heal like any other bone fracture. The downside to this procedure is that the knee is fused in a straight position, so

38

one will not be able to bend the knee, nor be able to do all functions that require knee bending. Pain, however, will be eliminated.

Tips

➢   *If you are overweight - lose weight.*

➢   *Use a cane, crutches, and/or other devices to protect your joint. These can be shoe inserts, walkers and splints.*

➢   *Put mobile shower heads in your bathroom. This way you do not have to move around in the shower. Bath seats and grab bars on bathtubs are other helpful additions.*

➢   *Do not carry heavy loads.*

➢   *Do not overuse your joints.*

➢   *Push on objects, instead of pulling them.*

➢   *Take your medications as prescribed by your doctor.*

➢   *Know how to use the RICE method at home by yourself.*

➢   *Strengthen your joints by exercising regularly.*

2) Knee rheumatoid arthritis

The exact cause of rheumatoid arthritis (RA) of the knee is unknown. Medical researchers, however, suspect that it only occurs in a susceptible individual after a trigger factor initiates an immune response. RA of the knee is the third most prevalent arthritis of the knee, affecting approximately 1.3 million people in the United States. This disease often begins slowly; symptoms may be just knee joint fatigue. Years after this long-term complaint is when other symptoms become apparent. RA of the knee may not only be of the knee, since RA is a systemic disease which affects multiple joints and other connective tissues of the body.

Knee RA affects anyone, at any age, even infants, but ages between 40 and 60 dominate. One predictor, however, is being of the female gender, since 75% of all cases affect women.

a) Knee RA development

Unlike OA, which results from the 'wear and tear' of the knee articulating cartilage, RA has a different development mechanism altogether. Knee RA is a chronic autoimmune disease in which an immune response is initiated to attack the tissues of the knee joint. In RA of the knee, a chronic inflammation is always present with episodes of flares and remission. The disease usually affects symmetrical joints in an ascending or descending fashion. For instance, one knee joint may be affected at the beginning, then after several months or even years, the other knee joint becomes symptomatic.

The immune system is made up of a complex organization of cells (lymphocytes) and antibodies designed to fight any foreign bodies that invade the body. An immune response is therefore the body's way of fighting infection. However, in knee RA, infection is absent, yet still a defective response is initiated against an individual's own tissue. This response does not attack tissues of the knee joint only, but general body tissues and organs. Because it affects multiple tissues of the body and organs, knee RA as an individual entity may actually be nonexistent. The collective term used is rheumatoid disease or rheumatoid arthritis.

b) Pathological picture of knee RA

Rheumatoid arthritis of the knee has 4 distinguished stages. These stages occur gradually, though the disease is almost always progressive.

Stage 1 - the period at which the immune system invents a defective response to attack own its body tissues. Besides an immune response being initiated, the condition in itself is asymptomatic. However, medical tests such as an ESR can be done, and CRP and rheumatoid factor (RF) may be detected in the blood. Their presence in blood can be detected years before the first diagnosis, though not in every case.

Stages 2 - early changes within the knee joint appear due to chronic inflammation. These changes include cellular infiltrates that float in the synovial fluid. The synovial membrane thickens and becomes inflamed, which is known as synovitis. Due to its hypertrophy, the synovium also begins to produce a lot of synovial fluid. Therefore, swelling of the knee due to joint effusion may occur at this stage. Blood vessels become congested, and many new vessels form so that the knee becomes hot or warm to touch. Arthralgia is the most prevalent complaint in all sufferers, although the joint in itself is still intact.

Stage 3 - as the inflammation persists, the vast cells in the joint release enzymes, which greatly contribute to eroding the knee joint tissues. Tendons get tenosynovitis, which with daily use may lead to partial or total tendon tears. The articular cartilage is destroyed, and the smooth function of the joint is disturbed. The joint is basically destroyed.

Stage 4 - articular cartilage disruption results in bones rubbing against each other during movement. A progressive joint imbalance occurs, disfiguring the normal knee joint appearance.

At this stage, the disease is irreversible, and treatment plans are centered on pain relief and maintaining joint stability. Artificial knee replacements may be the only way out.

c) Risk factors of rheumatoid disease

Certain factors increase the probability of any one individual developing RA of the knee in their lifetime. These factors are listed below:

Genetic susceptibility - the fact that knee RA affects people who have first-degree relatives that also suffer from RA suggests a hereditary trait. Studies that were carried out in patients of RA showed a genetic association of the human leukocytic antigen (HLA-DR4). This means that any person who has the gene codes for HLA-DR4 may at some point in their life suffer from RA.

Gender – females of 40-60 years of age are the dominating group in RA diagnosis. Women are 3 times more at risk of suffering RA compared to men.

Rheumatoid factor - if detected in blood, one may later on be diagnosed as having RA. Rheumatoid factor (RF) is an antibody against immunoglobulin G of the body. However, its absence in blood does not rule out the diagnosis of RA.

Concomitant autoimmune diseases - people who are already suffering from any other autoimmune disease, e.g. SLE, are at a greater risk of developing RA.

Cigarette smoking - is associated with development of RA. Studies have also shown that the RA that develops in smokers is more severe than it otherwise would be.

Stress - stressful life events like divorce or the death of a loved one are common findings in people who suffer from RA.

History of food allergies may be noted in some sufferers.

d) Signs and symptoms

Like any other type of arthritis, knee RA has signs and symptoms that are specific in its progression. These symptoms help to differentiate rheumatoid disease from any other type of arthritis. However, it is safer to have a doctor diagnose the condition accurately than to believe in its presence and/or to self-diagnose. Self-diagnosis can be dangerous. Since in the early stages of knee RA the condition can be somewhat reversible, one wouldn't want to miss this window of opportunity. In other cases, a more immediate disease like septic arthritis can be missed, only to be realized later after the joint has been severely destroyed, with bone abscesses of the thigh bone or shin bone.

Symptoms may appear as episodes, which are called flares. Flares occur when RA of the knee is active. Inflammatory processes at this point take an acute presentation, over an already existing chronic inflammatory picture. The flares stay for a long period of time on the very first episode; however, with time their duration shortens. Remission may last a year or more, although some joint fatigue or discomfort will still be present.

Knee joint pain, swelling, warmth and tenderness are the main patient complaints. Knee joint stiffness in the morning that lasts for over 45 minutes is typical. The stiffness gradually disappears as one tends to bend and straighten the knee repeatedly to loosen this stiffness. Knee ligaments become lax, giving way of the knee during movement points at joint instability. Weather changes also tend to affect patients with RA. The cold and extremely hot weather can be a trigger factor for a flare-up to occur. Most patients lose weight, maybe because of the immune suppression that occurs in rheumatoid disease.

During flare-ups, fever, sweating and general body weakness may accompany signs that support rheumatoid disease to be a systemic condition. The knee range of motion may be limited, and patients complain of more pain when the joint is moved. The gait of affected individuals has a limp, which is known as antalgic gait. This type of walking is noticed in people who have joint pain. In a normal step, there are 2 phases identified; the stance phase and the swing phase. The stance phase occupies 60% of a single step cycle. It involves the foot touching the ground up until the foot is ready to be lifted off the ground again. The swing phase occupies 40% of the step cycle, from the point when the foot takes off from the ground to when it touches the ground. In antalgic gait, a patient shortens the stance phase, which is the time that the knee supports most of the weight of the body. In other words, the patient unknowingly changes the way they walk to try and avoid further injury to the joint. General body fatigue, muscle pain, numbness and tingling sensations in fingers and toes are other reported signs.

Knee RA often has additional locations. The condition in itself may actually start with other joints before coming to the knee. This is true, more often than not, for the joints of the hands and feet. In other cases, however, RA will start by affecting a single large joint such as the knee.

Associated conditions

**Tarsal tunnel syndrome and/or carpal tunnel syndrome - ** in rheumatoid disease, general body connective tissues are hypertrophied due to chronic inflammation. This causes ligaments and tendons of the body to thicken. Most peripheral nerves pass in tunnels that are made from ligamentous tissue, such that when they thicken in RA, nerve passages become narrow and compress the nerves. This is why a lot of RA patients develop nerve compression syndromes. The main signs that they experience include numbness and tingling of the fingers and toes, a restless sensation that requires them to shake their feet or hands for temporary relief.

Nodules - painless lumps may appear under the skin. They occur mostly in areas of frequent pressure like the elbow.

Eyes - another frequently affected organ, the sclera (white part of the eye) can become inflamed, resulting in dry eyes, pain and reduced eye sight.

Blood vessels - may become inflamed anywhere in the body, which is called vasculitis. Symptoms depend on location of the vessels.

Inflammation in the chest cavity may cause pleuritis (inflammation of the chest lining) and pericarditis (inflammation of the heart's outer layer of connective tissue). These may result in easy fatigue, persistent cough, breathlessness, and susceptibility to development of pneumonia.

e) Diagnosis of knee RA

The diagnosis of RA of the knee is difficult, since many diseases mimic its presentation. It is also important to determine the progression of the disease as benign (type 1) or aggressive (type 2).

The presence of several of the following leads to a high suspicion of RA of the knee:

1) Morning stiffness of the knee, which lasts for 45 minutes or more, presenting for at least 6 weeks

2) Swelling on bilateral knee joints

3) The presence of nodules under the skin

4) Rheumatoid factor detected in blood, and/or anti-citrullinated protein antibodies.

5) Swelling of wrist, hand, or finger joints for at least 6 weeks, or the ankle, foot or toes.

6) The deviation of the hand towards the small finger (ulnar deviation)

These are the main, specific findings in patients with knee RA.

Besides a complete patient history and a thorough knee examination, a physician orders medical tests that help to diagnose. Medical tests that are done for rheumatoid arthritis of the knee increase the probability that RA is actually the diagnosis; however, on their own the diagnosis is not definite.

Elevated ESR, CRP, and increased white blood cells, especially lymphocytes, suggest the presence of an inflammatory process.

Rheumatoid factor presence is about 80% specific in RA patients; however, it can also be found in patients with other diseases. RF detection is an indicator of a type 2 RA course of disease.

Knee joint X-rays can show soft tissue swelling, synovitis, periarticular osteoporosis and arthritic changes, often reduced joint space; however, they are normal in early knee RA.

Ultrasound, in particular quantitative ultrasound (QUS), is somewhat reliable in monitoring joint inflammation. QUS is used to detect osteoporosis. This use is important in detecting osteoporosis of the hands, which is an early sign of RA.

Synovial fluid aspirate - in knee RA, synovial fluid is rich in cellular components and debris, which is an indicator of chronic inflammation.

f) Differential diagnosis of knee RA

Osteoarthritis (OA)

- In OA the knee joint is less inflamed.

 - Affects above-60-year-olds.

- Located on a single, large joint, e.g. knee.

- Rarely has a systemic involvement.

- Plain X-rays show osteophytes, bony spurs, reduced joint space, subchondral cysts and sclerosis.

Gout and pseudo gout

- Often starts in one joint

- Specific medical history (see gout arthritis of the knee)

- Detection of crystals in knee aspirate

- Plain X-rays show tophi (accumulations of crystals to form a lump), and tendon calcifications.

- High uric acid levels in blood

Differential diagnosis should be done for other autoimmune disorders like SLE and scleroderma. Other types of arthritis such as reactive arthritis, Reiter's syndrome, infectious arthritis, viral arthritis and septic arthritis should be ruled out. Also, other immune suppressing diseases like leukemia, AIDS and cancer should be eliminated from the diagnosis. After all this, when an actual RA of the knee diagnosis is made, treatment should be initiated.

g) Treatment of knee RA

First and foremost, patients should be educated on the developmental mechanisms of knee RA and how to assist themselves in reducing pain and other symptoms. Like in OA, the RICE method is an initial home remedy that anyone can master with no difficulties. Non-steroidal anti-inflammatory drugs (NSAIDs) can be bought as over-the-counter medicines for pain relief. However, the mainstay of treatment in RA of the knee is suppressing an overactive immune system. A specific group of drugs called DMARDs, standing for disease-modifying anti-rheumatic drugs, is often a good choice as they reduce both the symptoms and the rate at which the disease progresses. Methotrexate is an example; it acts by counteracting the immune response attacking the joint. Also, sulfasalazine is another example. The second group of DMARDs consists of biological modifiers. These include rituximab and Enbrel. However, one has to read their side effects carefully and make a well-informed choice. For example, Enbrel has a black box of infections that can occur as side effects.

B-cells and T-cells are subdivisions of cells that are called lymphocytes, whose major role is in the immune system. B-cell and T-cell inhibitors are a group of immunosuppressive drugs that target these cells. Cortisone shots are also in use for pain relief in knee RA, and so are hyaluronic acid injections. Tumor necrosis factor (TNF) inhibitors are another group of drugs used for treatment of RA of the knee.

Availability of all these medications on insurance depends on the insurance company. For example, some private insurance companies can only approve TNF inhibitors after one has tried Prednisone, Methotrexate and Arava. Funny enough, some medical insurance companies just require a prescription for the TNF inhibitors. Most patients, however, prefer methotrexate because it has been around for long, and its side effects, if compared to TNF inhibitors, are minimal.

Gold injections are also used for treatment of RA, e.g. Myochrisine, which is injected into muscles. Gold injections are among the original medicines that have been used in RA treatment. They have been on the market for over 75 years. It is not entirely clear how these medications work, but they are known to modify the immune response, thus they exhibit anti-inflammatory properties. Gold injections have also been condemned for kidney complications; therefore their use requires close monitoring. Besides injections, tablets are also available.

Alternative methods of treatment such as acupuncture and magnetic pulse therapy may also be implemented; however, they have limited research on outcomes.

Exercises and physiotherapy are recommended and are to be described under the physiotherapy topic.

Surgical procedures include synovectomy, which is a procedure done by a surgeon to remove the thick synovium. It can be done as an arthroscopic procedure or as open surgery. However, keyhole surgery of arthroscopy is preferred because it gives few complications and is cosmetically accepted. Total knee joint replacement surgery is often performed as a last resort, for severely destroyed joints.

Tips

➢ *Avoid stretching the knee joint when inflammation is active, stick to gentle passive and active movements, adequate to maintain FROM.*

➢ *Short exercises, e.g. 10-minute duration, for several times a day are preferred to one long session.*

➢ *Learn the RICE method, and always keep a supply of NSAIDs in a safe place in your home.*

➢ *To avoid stiffness of the knee joint, change position frequently.*

➢ *Research more on RA of the knee from many sources, e.g. educative books, the Internet and discussions with your doctor.*

3) Gout arthritis of the knee

a) What is gout?

In a normal individual, body waste products from a lot of biochemical processes in all body systems are excreted by the kidneys as urine, through the skin as sweat, and/or are detoxified in the liver. The metabolism of proteins, deoxyribonucleic acid (DNA) and ribonucleic acids (RNA) produce purines, which are converted to uric acid during their excretion. In gout arthritis, uric acid is produced in large quantities, and/or is excreted with limitations, so that its levels in blood increase significantly. To maintain the blood acidity on check, this extra uric acid is removed from the blood, where it enters into joints. Uric acid in joints crystallizes to form monosodium urate crystals.

The presence of these crystals in the knee joint is the main pathological change that substantiates the diagnosis of knee gout arthritis. However, since uric acid circulates in blood, generally the monosodium urate crystals can be formed in multiple joints.

b) Epidemiology of gout arthritis of the knee

In under-65s, men have 4 times more risk of developing gout arthritis than women, and in over-65s, the risk is still high in men, but drops to 3 times more likely. Black men are affected with gout at twice the rate of their white counterparts. There are several hospital admissions that occur due to gout yearly, however, no cost studies have been reported on the burden that it has on the economy. Gout affects about 1-2 people per every 100, and yearly in the United States about 1 million people are diagnosed with this disease.

c) Developmental stages of knee gout arthritis

Gout arthritis of the knee can be visualized in 4 stages. These stages are:

Stage 1 - an individual at this stage has hyperuricemia (a high blood content of uric acid), however, symptoms are absent. The disease is not evident, but is in progression as monosodium urate crystals form and deposit in tissues, resulting in damage.

Stage 2 - when accumulating crystals cause an inflammatory response in the knee for the first time, stage 2 is marked. The knee joint is symptomatic at this stage, with pain, heat, and swelling that lasts for days to weeks. However, in general, gout may often begin with pain of the big toe before it attacks a large joint like the knee, which is called podagra. Podagra may be a late presentation in a patient who is already suffering from knee gout arthritis. Testing for uric acid in the blood of affected people may be surprisingly normal. However, signs and symptoms lead to a high suspicion of the disease and a physician then orders further tests.

Stage 3 - the flare-up on stage 2 subsides, and the disease enters into remission. In the background, more monosodium urate crystals get deposited in the joint and tissues of the body, causing further damage. As the disease progresses, remissions last for a shorter duration.

Stage 4 - the accumulating crystals result in a permanent, chronic inflammation of the knee joint, hence a chronic gout arthritis. The joint becomes sore and achy. Huge lumps of crystals known as tophi form around the joint, which is also seen in the elbow and the ear.

d) Risk factors to knee GA development

There are several risk factors that can predispose an individual to developing gout arthritis of the knee.

1) **Gender** – the male gender is affected 3-4 times more than the female gender.

2) **Age** - rarely are children and young adults affected; people between 40-50 years of age dominate, with the peak age at 75 years old.

3) **Genetics** - in approximately 20% of cases, a genetic association has been linked to GA of the knee.

4) **Diet** - excessive alcohol intake increases the risk of developing GA, since it prevents uric acid excretion. Large quantities of meat (game), sea foods and fructose-based drinks have been shown to be contributory to the disease condition in 12% of cases.

5) **Medical conditions** that reduce uric acid excretion like kidney diseases, and metabolic states that increase the production of uric acid and/or reduce its excretion are linked to GA development.

6) **Medications** that eliminate fluid from the body such as diuretics and those used for treatment of edema increase the risk of GA.

Additional risks include lead exposure and frequent episodes of dehydration.

e) Diagnosis of knee GA

Knee joint aspirate examination is the gold standard of diagnosing GA of the knee. A doctor, under sterile conditions, and by using a needle, aspirates some synovial fluid from the knee. This fluid is then put on a glass slide and is viewed under a microscope. The presence of shiny urate crystals is confirmatory. However, the absence of these crystals from the joint aspirate does not exclude the diagnosis. Joint aspirate may also be taken to the laboratory for culturing to exclude any infection of the knee joint.

A blood test for uric acid can be checked, though often their results can be misleading. An individual with a positive uric acid test may not be suffering from gout, while one with signs and symptoms of GA may test negative for uric acid.

A plain X-ray film will show arthritis joint space changes with at times tophi.

Otherwise an experienced doctor may diagnose GA of the knee from the clinical presentation of the disease, patient complaints, and physical examination findings.

f) Symptoms and signs of GA

- Presence of urate crystals in joint aspirate.

- Several attacks (episodes or flares) of acute joint arthritis.

- Arthritis where when active even for 24 hours, the knee joint becomes swollen, very painful, tender, hot, and hyperaemic (red).

- One joint is affected, e.g. knee, though in the elderly the picture may be different, affecting several joints and hence being mistaken for any other type of arthritis.

- Hyperuricemia.

- Pain may specifically start at night.

- Reduced ROM of the joint.

- Itching joints, and peeling off of skin around the knee joint as a flare subsides.

- Presence of tophi on other joints, e.g. the elbow and hands.

- Bursitis of the knee (pre-patellar bursa) is a common finding.

g) Differential diagnosis
RA

OA

Septic arthritis

HIV infection

Diabetes

Kidney infection

Pseudogout - presents like gout arthritis of the knee. The major difference is in the type of crystals that accumulate in the joint. Calcium pyrophosphate dehydrate crystals are deposited in the knee joint in pseudogout.

h) Treatment of knee GA

After the diagnosis of gouty knee has been made, a treatment plan can be made together with your doctor. The initial aim is to relieve pain and inflammation of the joint. After an attack resolves, treatment is then directed at preventing another attack, the progression of the disease, and to maintain the knee joint function optimally.

Though without treatment gout flare-ups resolve on their own after several weeks, one can speed up recovery by a number of ways.

1) **The RICE method** is started as soon as an episode of gout arthritis is evident.

2) **NSAIDs** can help reduce pain, if started as soon as the symptoms appear. Aspirin is also an NSAID, but should not be used for a gouty knee due to its action of rapidly increasing uric acid levels in blood. Therefore, when used, aspirin worsens an attack of gout. Before using any NSAIDs, run it past your doctor for advice.

3) **Corticosteroids** can be taken as tablets, or injections into the joint; however, a doctor should always consent before its use.

The main focus of treatment of a gouty knee is to prevent excess uric acid in the blood, and the formation of urate crystals. Some specific drugs are used in the treatment of gout due to the fact that they affect uric acid concentrations in the blood and urate crystal development; such drugs include Colchicine and Allopurinol.

4) **Colchicine** tablets can be taken to reduce the buildup of urate in joints. The use of colchicine should be approved by your doctor. Any allergies are to be reported before its use, and

simultaneous alcohol intake decreases its effectiveness. Its use in people with liver and kidney diseases may be contraindicated. Side effects of this drug include nausea and diarrhea.

5) **Allopurinol** is yet another drug used to treat hyperuricemic syndrome and chronic gout. Allopurinol reduces uric acid production. It's used during remission to manipulate the disease course and progression. However, its use during a gout attack is controversial as it is said to worsen the condition. Like any other medication, Allopurinol is dispensed on prescription.

6) **Diet control** is a supportive regimen in gout arthritis treatment. Reduce foods that lead to formation of purines, e.g. fish, spinach, and asparagus.

7) **Surgeries** often performed for gout arthritis of the knee are;

- The removal of tophi for cosmetic reasons.

- Arthroscopic washing up of the joint to remove some crystals.

8) **Physiotherapy** of the knee is a must, and is discussed under the physiotherapy section.

Tips

➤　　*Avoid excess weight loss over a short period of time.*

➤　　*If you are taking any medications for any other disease, ask your doctor to review them for their chances of worsening a gouty knee, e.g. heart disease medications.*

➤　　*Take a lot of vitamin C, as citrus fruits or supplements. Studies have shown that 5,500 mg of Vitamin C in a day can reduce the risk of GA by at least 45%.*

➢　*Avoid drinking excess alcohol and fructose-sweetened drinks.*

➢　*Exercise and stretches help maintain the joint function, strength and stability.*

4) Septic arthritis of the knee

The term 'septic' is used in reference to an infection. Septic arthritis is also known as infectious arthritis or bacterial arthritis. Septic arthritis of the knee is therefore a type of arthritis that occurs due to infection in the knee joint. Infections can be of several kinds, depending on the infective agent, and different age groups may be affected by different causative agents, e.g. gonococcal arthritis in the sexually active age group. In septic arthritis (SA) of the knee, staphylococcal and streptococcal infections dominate.

a) Causes of SA of the knee

There are many ways in which bacteria can find their way into the knee joint. The first way is through a direct inoculation/introduction into the joint by surgery, trauma, and/or simple procedures like joint aspiration if they are done under a non-sterile setup. The second way is that somewhere else in the body, there may be an infective process going on, e.g. an ear infection, and bacteria from this site are transported through the bloodstream to the joint, which is known as the hematogenous pathway. In other cases, bacteria enter the knee joint from a nearby infection e.g. osteomyelitis of the femur. However it happens, infectious arthritis of the knee is an emergency.

b) Pathological processes in a knee with SA

After an infective agent enters the knee joint, an inflammatory response is initiated as the body tries to fight off infection. The severity of the host response is somewhat determined by the host susceptibility to an infection. Host susceptibility to knee infection is enhanced by immunosuppression. Factors that suppress immunity include malnutrition, other chronic conditions such as diabetes and HIV/AIDS, vascular disorders, trauma and long-term corticosteroid use. This means that in people with the aforementioned immunosuppressive conditions, the risk of developing SA of the knee is greater and a severe form often develops.

Unlike RA, which is a systemic condition that affects several joints, SA rarely affects multiple joints at a time. SA in general occurs in about 20,000 people per year in the United States, European figures are similar, and the knee is affected in 50% of these cases. The incidence of SA in individuals who had a prosthetic joint replacement range between 1.5-2.5% for first-time procedures, while reaching as high as 20% for revised procedures.

Stage 1 - soon after the joint gets infected, a systemic response appears where pain and fever are the leading symptoms. The synovium of the joint gets inflamed and thickens, producing an increased amount of synovial fluid in response. The knee joint is swollen due to the synovial effusion, which soon changes to pus because of the ongoing infection.

Treatment initiation at this stage prevents further joint destruction, which is usually very rapid.

Stage 2 - without any treatment intervention, pus and the infection erode the articular cartilage. There are two ways by which this erosion occurs: bacterial toxins and enzymes act directly on the cartilage or the synovial cells release proteolytic enzymes to try and kill the bacteria. Instead, these enzymes also attack cartilage tissue, thereby destroying the joint.

Vascular compromise may also be present at this stage, which will cause bone infarction and necrosis. In a child with SA of the knee, the destruction is severe, so severe that the growth plates of the femur and the tibia can be completely eroded.

If treatment is still not initiated at this stage, a knee abscess with a sinus forms and further development of osteomyelitis is inevitable.

If adequate treatment is given, depending on the stage at which it is initiated, the knee infection may completely resolve with knee joint structure survival. However, joint fibrosis, fusion, and permanent deformity often result.

c) Who is at risk of developing knee SA

Anyone can be affected with knee SA; however, certain individuals have an increased risk of its development.

1) People with open knee wounds or open trauma of the knee are at a greater risk.

2) Young children and the elderly.

3) Immunosuppressed individuals.

4) Individuals who are already suffering from one form of arthritis, e.g. RA or OA. If knee SA develops over another non-infectious arthritis, its diagnosis can be very difficult, resulting in a possible late diagnosis.

5) People who have had an artificial joint replacement.

6) Street drug abusers.

7) People on chemotherapy.

d) Signs and symptoms of infectious arthritis of the knee

- Pain on any slight knee joint movement is the main complaint. In children they refuse to use the joint, which is called pseudoparalysis.

- A tender swelling develops over the knee joint.

- Hyperaemia (redness) over the knee joint is typical.

- General body malaise and fever are additional signs. In children, fever may be very high, enough to cause a febrile seizure.

- A single joint is affected.

- Bacteraemia and sepsis are common findings, which are reasons why the presentation of acute knee SA is serious to grave.

- SA of the knee has an acute presentation, which is reported within 1-2 days. Because the clinical picture of a sufferer is usually serious, most patients seek treatment early. This, however, is not so in some knee joint infections, especially TB, which is chronic and occurs slowly over several months to even a year.

- Risky findings to the development of knee SA are very common.

e) Differential diagnosis

- Other types of knee arthritis, e.g. RA and OA.

- Reactive arthritis, e.g. postgonoccocal arthritis.

- Viral arthritis

- Knee gout arthritis is the closest diagnosis to SA of the knee in presentation. Careful evaluation during diagnosis is necessary.

f) Diagnosis

1) Routine FBC reveals elevated white blood cells, especially neutrophils, which is known as neutrophilia.

2) Inflammatory markers such as ESR and CRP are also greatly increased. Though all these are not specific for diagnosing SA of the knee, a positive test assists in confirming the diagnosis. CRP and ESR can also be used as markers for checking the effectiveness of treatment. If proper treatment is initiated, these markers are expected to decrease over time, so weekly testing is done, and then after 2-3 weeks the results are compared.

3) Synovial fluid aspiration is the top ranking standard of diagnosing knee SA. If pus is aspirated from the joint, one is a step ahead of diagnosing infectious arthritis of the knee, though this on its own is inadequate to substantiate the disease. Further medical tests are required for adequate treatment planning.

Joint aspirate is taken to the laboratory for testing. One common finding is leukocytosis (increased white blood cells). This synovial fluid is also cultured on a medium to allow the causative agent to grow, and then a specific antibiogram is concluded.

Often, when all these lab works are going on behind the scenes, the patient is started on intravenous broad spectrum antibiotics blindly, to prevent a delay in treatment. When the lab results become available, as to the specific infectious agent together with its antibiogram, a specific effective antibiotic is started. If the medication that had been empirically initiated is also on the antibiogram, a replacement is not required and that same drug is continued to make a complete dose.

Knee joint aspirate is also checked under the microscope for crystals, to rule out an infected gouty knee or an infection over pseudogout.

After gram staining, it is important to have other stains done on the joint aspirate. A disease like tuberculosis of the knee is often diagnosed this way.

When fungi are the probable causative agents, a synovial tissue biopsy is the main method of diagnosis.

In severely sick individuals, who are suspected of having sepsis, a blood culture is indicated.

Viral infections of the knee joint will require further tests of viral DNA or RNA testing, where polymerase chain reaction is the standard diagnostic test, or consecutive immunological viral antibody titer checks.

In addition to laboratory tests, imaging tests are a must. Plain X-rays are available in most medical centers, and they are cheap to almost everyone. Therefore, they are often the initial imaging test done. On X-ray, cartilage destruction, joint effusion, surrounding soft tissue swelling, bone infection, reduced joint space with fusion (ankylosis) of the joint, and sclerosis may be noted. Not necessarily all of these features are seen. Their presence depends on the severity and the stage of knee bacterial arthritis. These X-ray changes, however, require an experienced eye to pick out the presence of an infection; otherwise one might think of any other form of arthritis.

Ultrasound is helpful, especially in children who are often symptomatic, but have normal knee joints on plain X-rays. An ultrasound will show dense synovial fluid which is consistent with pus, and may also be used to guide a diagnostic needle for joint aspiration, or a treatment needle to tap off excess synovial fluid/pus.

A CT scan is an excellent diagnostic imaging technique for bone diseases, including abscesses, and osteomyelitis, though it can be expensive. Its availability is limited to specialized centers and major hospitals.

MRI is yet another expensive imaging technique, whose availability is also limited, although its accuracy and precision is excellent. Knee joint effusion, tendon and ligament injuries, cartilage destruction, and vascular compromise are clearly visualized by MRI. It is important, however, to note that an MRI machine produces a high magnetic field current, hence its use is contraindicated in patients with metal components in their bodies, e.g. artificial heart valves and replaced joints.

g) Treatment of knee SA

First and foremost, pain elimination is one of the targets of treatment. Analgesics like diclofenac and ibuprofen can be bought over-the-counter. Since most patients run a fever and are dehydrated, intravenous (IV) fluid therapy is also necessary. These IV fluids include Ringer's lactate and normal saline; however, dextrose normal saline and 5% glucose solution are good options for children who tend to lose their appetite when they get sick with knee SA.

The knee joint requires splinting as a way of immobilizing the joint to reduce pain. Temporary use of crutches, a cane or a walker may be beneficial.

Early IV antibiotics are a must. They are to be started as soon as the provisional diagnosis of infectious arthritis of the knee has been made. A very important thing to note is that antibiotics should be given after all fluid samples for laboratory tests have been collected, e.g. blood and joint aspirate. This is to maximize the efficiency of the lab test results. The initial choice of antibiotics for use as an empirical treatment is based on a high suspicion of the most probable causative agent. This probability is learned by most physicians during medical school and through experience. In general, staphylococcus aureus is the culprit infectious agent. However, some discrepancies arise with age, e.g. in babies a streptococcal infection. Penicillin and cephalosporin antibiotic groups are the most used medications for knee infection blind therapy.

Evacuating pus from the joint is also a great benefit, and this procedure is done under anesthesia. After aspirating the joint is complete, irrigation is done using warm, normal saline solution, and a drainage tube is left in place for 48-72 hours. In severe cases or cases where the aspirate is too thick, several joint irrigations may be necessary for 2-4 days. This is usually done by means of using arthroscopy; otherwise an open surgery (arthrotomy) is suggested if the first option fails. If the infection has occurred in a joint that has had an artificial replacement, in almost all the cases the implants have to be removed.

As soon as the patient is not in so much pain and is on the way to recovery, physiotherapy of the joint should be performed. This physiotherapy is aimed at maintaining knee joint mobility. Sadly, this is only possible when treatment has been initiated in the early developmental stages of SA, otherwise joint fusion in late developmental stages may be inevitable. To assist such a case, applying a cast on the lower limb for several weeks will help the knee joint to fuse in at least a functional position.

h) Complications and prognosis

When treatment is initiated determines the long-term outlook on the disease. In stage 1- the infection usually clears up with no complications. Stage 2 also may clear without any complications, however, pus often causes rapid destruction of cartilage, and after resolution patients usually complain of chronic knee pain with some reduced mobility. In the latest stages, a straight fused leg results. Though walking function will be preserved, one will not be able to bend the knee again (like in an arthrodesis). If growth plates in children are destroyed, leg length discrepancies and disability result.

Tips

➤ *Educate yourself on the condition by reading books, searching the Web, and asking your physician. Joining health discussion groups can also help you to appreciate that you are not alone - the treatment options that are working for others, and the ones that are a waste of time.*

➤ *Positive thinking, eating well, and sleeping for 8 hours or more can improve your mood.*

➤ *Live a stress-free life; pamper yourself - for instance, a warm shower before bed can help release tense muscles, thereby making your sleep bliss. Consider employing a certified masseuse who can give you a few sessions during the week.*

➤ *Always protect your joint when it's still sore. Rest and splints are useful.*

➤ *Maintain activity by doing ROM exercises and knee muscle strengthening exercises (only when ready to initiate strengthening exercises).*

5) Post-traumatic arthritis of the knee

The term 'post-trauma' defines itself. Post-traumatic arthritis of the knee is inflammation of a knee that has had previous injury. Injury to the knee joint can be open or closed. Open injuries, besides causing post-traumatic arthritis, may also cause bacterial arthritis. Injuries of the knee joint are frequent, especially in this current era, where a lot of people are participating in sporting activities to lose weight or maintain their body size. Motor traffic accidents and falls are other contributory factors to knee injury.

At some point in the lifetime of a normal individual, arthritis of the knee develops slowly. However, after an injury, its development is faster depending on how severe the injury was. 12% of all OA occur due to previous trauma. The figures are approximated to be around 5.6 million in the United States.

a) How does injury cause post-traumatic arthritis of the knee

Reasons as to why trauma may cause arthritis years after injury are divided into direct and indirect reasons.

Direct reasons

1) Direct injury to the knee, e.g. fracture of the tibial plateau, may result in the articular surface splitting and/or chipping off. Cartilage is a type of connective tissue which has no regeneration power, so that an injury will heal with scar tissue. This scar tissue will result in adhesions forming in the knee joint. The functional strength of scar tissue is inferior to that of the original cartilage.

2) When the joint surface heals, the gap in articular cartilage, which is known as an intra-articular extension, creates an uneven joint surface. If treatment does not approximate fracture margins

accurately, there will be rubbing and grinding during movement, which predisposes the joint to arthritis.

3) The stabilizing components of the knee, ligaments and tendons may directly be injured by trauma. Their injury leads to knee joint instability and giving way during movement, which further injures the joint surface.

Indirect reasons

1) After trauma to one knee, the normal knee is used for movement with the help of crutches; this predisposes the uninjured knee to early arthritis as it carries more weight than usual.

2) When one gets knee trauma, a cast is usually applied to allow for fractures to heal. Temporary loss of mobility of the joint will result in joint stiffness after the cast is removed. This stiffness, together with other complications that arise due to immobilization, e.g. muscle atrophy, predisposes the knee to early arthritis.

3) After trauma, some free bony or cartilaginous chips float freely in the synovial fluid, which are called loose bodies. Loose bodies often result in locking and sticking of the knee joint during movement, which further injures the joint surface.

b) Symptoms of knee post-traumatic arthritis

Symptoms of post-traumatic knee arthritis include pain. This pain is dull in nature, which is irritating and annoying to most sufferers. However, as the disease progresses, the achy character of pain changes to become sharp and more severe. Swelling of the knee is yet another finding, which is worse after periods of inactivity, i.e. in the morning. Joint effusion, tenderness and stiffness are a triad which make sufferers dread taking the first step in the morning. After a few stretches, it gets a bit smoother. Increased activity leads to severe pain afterwards. In severe post-traumatic arthritis of the knee, there is reduced joint mobility and the knee joint is deformed.

c) *Diagnosing post-traumatic arthritis of the knee*

Everyone that has been diagnosed with post-traumatic arthritis of the knee has a history of knee trauma. Complete medical history taking is done by a doctor, physical examination and any other medical tests or imaging are performed. The diagnosis is made after the results of all these evaluations are reviewed.

d) *Treatment of knee post-traumatic arthritis*

It is unfortunate that post-traumatic arthritis cannot be prevented. One could say that avoiding injury will prevent this condition. It's easier said than done, as injuries occur when we least expect it. One could be coming from work at the end of the day and get involved in a car accident. To some extent we can prevent injury by following safety guidelines like not drinking and driving, fastening a seatbelt when in a car and maintaining speed limits. However, once injury has occurred, it's a race against time to the moment at which post-traumatic arthritis becomes symptomatic.

Symptoms of post-traumatic arthritis can be treated as follows:

1) Pain is managed by NSAIDs, e.g. aspirin or naproxen, ice packs, cortisone shots and a complete RICE regimen.

2) Knee support by orthotic devices increases knee joint stability during movement. Knee-ankle-foot orthosis (KAFO), knee braces and knee supports are examples of helpful devices used for post-traumatic arthritis. Crutches, canes or walkers may also be temporarily used to remove extra weight from an injured knee.

3) Combinations of glucosamine and chondroitin supplements, weight loss, physiotherapy, and occupational therapy are also implemented for treatment of knee arthritis resulting after trauma.

4) When conservative measures fail to improve the quality of life of a sufferer, an orthopedic specialist may perform surgery. Surgical procedures that can be done depend on the severity of knee joint destruction by post-traumatic arthritis.

Partial and total knee joint replacements are frequent procedures, which over the years have increased in their rate of success. Knee joint replacement involves an orthopedic specialist removing the articular surface of the femur and tibia, and then reapplying similar, though artificial components of the knee joint. Knee joint replacement requires one to be well-informed before the procedure is carried out.

6) General overview facts of knee arthritis

In any one form of the 5 types of knee arthritis discussed, there are several kinds of specialists who can accurately diagnose and manage knee arthritis. Orthopedic surgeons, rheumatologists, family physicians, rehabilitation and sports medicine specialists are the best options. Occupational therapists, masseuses and chiropractors are the perfect supportive team to the main doctors.

Arthritis of the knee is an incurable, progressive disease, regardless of the type. From our understanding of developmental mechanisms of all knee arthritis, certain treatment options are almost always supportive, e.g. diet. However, patient comfort and quality of life can be improved by various treatment approaches that we have already discussed. The good thing is that knee arthritis, in general, is not a lethal disease, although a reduced life expectancy has been reported.

7) Addition 1 - Reactive arthritis

Reactive arthritis, like any other arthritis, is inflammation of a joint, and in the context of this book, of the knee joint. The term "reactive" means that a reaction is occurring in the joint due to something, most often an infection in another location of the body. The inflammation in a joint due to reactive arthritis is accompanied by the usual signs and symptoms of inflammation which include pain, tenderness, redness and swelling. However, a specific association in reactive arthritis symptoms is inflammation of the eye (conjunctivitis) and inflammation of the urinary tract (urethritis). Reactive arthritis is also classified as a seronegative spondyloarthropathy. Seronegative spondyloarthropathies is a group of diseases that cause generalized inflammation in the body, an example being ankylosing spondylosis of the spine.

a) What causes reactive arthritis?

Reactive arthritis is usually triggered by venereal diseases of the urinary system, e.g. gonorrhea. This is why reactive arthritis is at times called genitourinary reactive arthritis. Reactive arthritis may also result after an infection of the gastrointestinal tract (GIT), e.g. salmonella, and as such reactive arthritis can be called gastrointestinal reactive arthritis. Diseases of the respiratory tract like tonsillitis may also play a role in its development.

When these infections attack the body, our immune system generates antibodies and other mechanisms to fight them off. One theory is that when the infectious agents are killed by the immune system, their debris float in the bloodstream, and by chance can be deposited in the tissues of the joints. This triggers a local inflammatory response within the joint, which then gives off symptoms of a reactive arthritis. The other theory says that some bacteria, e.g. streptococci, have an outer membrane which is made up of certain protein sequences that are recognized by the cells of our immune system as foreign. While in the body, the tissues of the joints exhibit a structural sequence similar to that of these bacteria, such that circulating antibodies attack the joints after signaling mechanisms portray them to be foreign.

Reactive arthritis begins 2-4 weeks after the named infections, and in most cases the infection would have already been resolved. Reactive arthritis may last for a couple of months - 3-6 months is the frequently reported case - and resolves completely in most cases. However, a small percentage of sufferers have been reported to have developed long-term arthritis after a reactive arthritis.

b) Who gets reactive arthritis?

Reactive arthritis often affects people between 20 and 40-years-old, with an epidemiological dominance of the male gender. This could be due to the fact that men are at a greater risk of developing urethral infections from sexually transmitted diseases (STDs). However, respiratory and gastrointestinal infections can affect anyone, making reactive arthritis a common disease.

Since reactive arthritis is a seronegative spondyloarthropathy, this group of joint diseases is connected to the human leukocytic antigen-B27 gene. About 1 in every 14 people in the U.K. have this gene, although it doesn't necessarily mean that all these individuals with the gene will suffer from reactive arthritis. It simply means that when a trigger infection affects this group of people, they are more susceptible to develop reactive arthritis. And also, studies have shown that people with a diagnosed reactive arthritis who test positive for the HLA-B27 gene suffer an abrupt and more serious form of the disease.

71

Individuals who are HIV-positive may also be at an increased risk of developing reactive arthritis. This could be due to the human immunodeficiency virus itself, or due to the antiretroviral drugs that are used in treating the disease.

c) *Epidemiology of reactive arthritis*

Reactive arthritis affects men and women alike, usually young adults. In a certain study which was done in Oregon and Minnesota, enteric reactive arthritis occurred at an incidence of 0.6-3.1 cases per 100,000 people. Chlamydial infection was estimated to cause the highest reactive arthritis, at 4-8% of all people with Chlamydia.

d) *Diagnosing reactive arthritis*

Unfortunately, no single test can confirm the diagnosis of reactive arthritis. However, your doctor can be highly suspicious if you have had certain infections in the previous weeks and are having symptoms on the knee joint and/or any other joint. Diagnosis of reactive arthritis is thus based on the clinical presentation after an infection. However, blood tests like ESR, CRP and FBC are often done as a routine checkup. Additional medical tests like X-rays may be performed for differentiating other causes of arthritis such as rheumatoid arthritis and gout.

Other medical investigations may be carried out depending on the type of trigger infection that you had or still have. These additional investigations can be stool analysis for gastrointestinal infections, urinalysis, and sputum for respiratory infections. You may be transferred to a genitourinary specialist for a checkup on sexually transmitted diseases. Since reactive arthritis is associated with conjunctivitis and urethritis, you may be referred for a medical evaluation by an ophthalmologist or urologist.

In a well-equipped facility, the HLA-B27 gene can be tested, although a positive test is not specific to a reactive arthritis diagnosis. A complete medical history, thorough medical examination, and medical tests are the only tools that can help a doctor to arrive at this diagnosis. Most doctors, however, sometimes find it difficult to make a reactive arthritis diagnosis, since no one specific test can aid them in making a 100% confirmation of disease presence. This could be a direction of clinical and medical research.

Ophthalmologists, gynecologists, urologists, orthopedic surgeons and physicians are the doctors who come across this disease most often in their careers, so much that they may be the most experienced in the treatment of reactive arthritis.

e) Signs and symptoms of reactive arthritis
Pain in one joint is usually the main complaint, although asymmetrical or multiple joints may be affected simultaneously. This pain appears a few days to several weeks after an infection.

Symptoms of the infection preceding the reactive arthritis often include diarrhea, abdominal cramps, fever and urethritis. Reactive arthritis also exhibits 2 forms of musculoskeletal affection: arthritis and enthesitis. Arthritis symptoms are of an acute origin, affecting joints of the upper extremity in half of the cases. The arthritis resolves in 6 months to 1 year. Enthesitis is inflammation around sites of ligament, tendon, and joint capsule insertions. Enthesitis is also called enthesopathy and it usually causes heel pain when the Achilles tendon insertion is affected. Pain, swelling and tenderness at insertion sites is typical.

Other manifestations that may appear are extra-articular. These include mouth ulcers, conjunctivitis, nail changes, skin lesions, heart manifestations, and systemic symptoms of fever, headache, weight loss and generalized weakness.

f) Treatment of reactive arthritis

There is no specific cure for reactive arthritis, but symptom-alleviating treatments are available.

- NSAIDs are used as pain medications, e.g. naproxen.

- Corticosteroid injections can be given intra-articular for temporary pain relief.

- Creams and lotions can be applied topically to soothe symptoms. Most of these creams are corticosteroid-based.

- Systemic glucocorticoids.

- Antibiotics.

- DMARDs and immunosuppressive drugs like methotrexate can also be implemented.

- Physiotherapy.

- The so-called 'biological' medications like tumor necrosis inhibitors may be beneficial too.

8) Addition 2 - Psoriatic arthritis

Psoriatic arthritis affects some individuals who suffer from psoriasis. Psoriasis is a dermatological condition which results in red plaques of scaly skin forming, usually on the joint flexures. Psoriasis is common in white people, affecting 1 in every 50. People aged between 15 and 40 years are often affected, though any age group can be affected. Psoriasis occurs in individuals that have a fast turnover of skin cells. The reasons as to why this occurs are not clear. This rapid turnover of skin results in flaky plaques forming on the top layer of skin and at times the scalp. Scalp psoriasis appears as if one has severe dandruff.

Genetics has been blamed for the fast rate of skin cell turnover, since psoriasis occurs in individuals whose family member suffered or is suffering from psoriasis. Certain factors also enhance psoriatic plaques, and these are infections, stress, some medications like NSAIDs, smoking, alcohol, sunlight and trauma.

Psoriasis is usually diagnosed by a dermatologist by the typical appearance of the psoriatic rash, though a skin biopsy may substantiate this diagnosis. Psoriasis is a persistent disease; however, in some individuals it can completely go away with time. Psoriasis symptoms can be controlled by moisturizers, steroid ointments, coal tar preparations, Vitamin D-based treatments, and phototherapy using ultraviolet B light (UVB).

1 person out of 10 individuals who suffer or have suffered from psoriasis will develop psoriatic arthritis. The psoriatic arthritis develops within 10 years after psoriasis first appears on the skin. However, in some people, it develops even several years later. Psoriatic arthritis can be mild, moderate and severe. In severe forms, deformity of the joints which leads to permanent disability occurs.

The diagnosis of psoriatic arthritis should be made by a doctor, for differentiation of psoriatic arthritis from other arthritis types is necessary. RA, OA and other arthritis forms affect psoriasis sufferers like any other person. Psoriatic arthritis affects any joint in the body, although certain clinical categories of its different presentations exist. These categories are as follows:

Asymmetrical oligoarticular arthritis - this category is common. It affects a few joints, below a count of 5, and often large joints like the knee with other small joints of the hands.

Symmetrical polyarthritis - several joints are affected, in identical locations. For instance, if the right knee is affected, the left knee will also be affected.

Distal interphalangeal joints - the joints of the fingers that are close to the nail bed are affected, although this form is rare.

Spondylitis - inflammation of the spinal vertebral joints and discs. It may or may not affect the sacroiliac joints (the articulation between the lower end of the spine and the pelvis).

Arthritis mutilans - this presentation of psoriatic arthritis results in finger and toe deformities that resemble mutilation, although this category is very rare.

a) Diagnosing psoriatic arthritis

Psoriatic arthritis diagnosis can only be made if one has previously suffered from psoriasis or is suffering from psoriasis. However, in a few individuals the arthritis symptoms appear years before skin lesions of psoriasis appear. Its diagnosis is made on suspicion by a medical doctor; however, medical tests can be done to differentiate other types of arthritis. Blood tests and X-rays are performed routinely.

b) Symptoms

Pain and stiffness are the most common joint symptoms. Stiffness is more apparent in the morning, and following periods of inactivity for several minutes to hours. Enthesis is also a common finding, where joint swelling and tenderness are its clinical findings. 'Sausage-shaped' fingers are common, as tendons in the fingers thicken due to inflammation. Skin changes due to psoriasis may be evident; these include flaky, red and white skin patches and dandruff.

c) Treatment of psoriatic arthritis

Treatment plans for psoriatic arthritis are aimed at reducing pain and joint stiffness. NSAIDs are good at easing joint pain. However, some individuals have reported worsening of their psoriasis after using NSAIDs. Consult with your doctor if such symptoms occur. Other painkillers like codeine and paracetamol may be used, though these do not exhibit anti-inflammatory properties. Intra-articular cortisone injections may also be helpful in reducing the inflammatory process during flare-ups, though one has to understand that these injections only give temporary pain relief and are not to be used more than 3 times in a single joint.

Treatment regimens of psoriatic arthritis are also aimed at preventing disease progression and DMARDs like sulfasalazine are used. DMARDs in psoriatic arthritis treatment do not have an immediate pain or inflammation response; however, their effects are appreciated after several months of use. Physiotherapy is implemented as prophylaxis to disability. Regular joint exercises, swimming and stationary biking are effective physio routines. Other treatment methods are directed at psoriatic skin lesions, the likes of emollients, special light therapy and lotions.

Chapter 4) Knee artificial joint replacement

Patients with severe knee arthritis could be candidates for knee replacement. Knee replacement is also known as knee arthroplasty. It involves the surgical removal of defective bones of the knee joint, and placement of artificial components. These artificial components could be metal alloys, polymers, and/or high grade plastics. There are several models that you and your doctor can choose from, depending on your body mass index (BMI), age, expected knee performance and your general well-being.

The surgery itself is a complex procedure that requires an orthopedic specialist to carefully remove the affected sections of the articulating bones, then shape the remaining bit to accurately accommodate an artificial component. In a partial knee replacement, only one bone of the articulating bones at the knee is replaced, while in total arthroplasty, all surfaces are replaced.

1) Things to consider before undergoing knee arthroplasty

Psychological readiness is required for one to pull through the process of having a knee replacement. Psychological readiness is achieved when you put all your worries, concerns, and fears to rest. Achieving this can be difficult, and requires a lot of effort on your part, and also your surgeon's. Here are some helpful tips which have been adopted from 'Arthritis of the hip and Knee' by Allen, Brander, M.D., and Stilberg, M.D.:

1) Educate yourself about knee replacement surgery, pre-operative requirements, and the processes that happen during the procedure, post-operative care, and possible complications that may occur. In short, map out all the pros and cons of having knee replacement surgery by using books, the Internet, and opinions from specialists that work closely with knee arthroplasty.

2) In your area, locate the best specialized center in this procedure. This is often an orthopedic unit, with specialized orthopedic surgeons. Once you find a good center, look for an experienced surgeon who is to become your doctor. Vice versa, this can be done by finding an experienced surgeon first, and then visiting the center at which they work. Centers that are located close to where you live have added advantages. But then again, an experienced surgeon is the main concern here. This is important because your surgeon is to become your pivot of treatment for many years to come. However, do not only consider experience in your choice. A specialist's qualities should include personality, and ethical approach to patient care.

3) Second opinions will put your concerns to rest if you have any doubts. Having 2 or more specialists agreeing on a concept reduces the chances of being mismanaged.

4) Plan ahead financially f you have no medical insurance. Time availability should also be checked, i.e. have your surgery when you will be free from other responsibilities. Consider the chances of family being available for support.

5) Gain perspective by talking to people who have already undergone knee joint replacement. These people can be located over the Internet in discussion groups, or you could ask your doctor to organize a few of his patients who consent to sharing their experiences with you.

6) Be involved in the planning of the procedure by playing your role, e.g. practicing using crutches, exercising daily, and checking with your doctor when you need clarification.

7) Be prepared for bedridden time, usually lasting up to 6 weeks. Conduct all your arrangements, business and chores before the procedure time arrives. This will also help reduce stress in the post-operative period.

8) Modify your home before you leave for the hospital, e.g. having bars placed in the bathtub or getting a mobile shower head or a raised toilet seat. When you are discharged from the hospital, your home environment is adaptive to your exact needs. This makes life easy.

9) Find a home nurse assistant and maybe also a housemaid, who will help you with house chores and medication taking when you get home. When the post-surgical wound is fresh, your nurse assistant may help by dressing it on a daily basis to prevent infection and to allow optimal wound healing. These 2 people are not a must; one could also communicate with his/her family members before the surgery is done. You could have your sibling over to your house, or you could go to theirs. A wife may ask support from her husband who can take a leave from work if the arrangement allows, and vice versa. A certified, skilled physiotherapist should also be arranged before surgery. Rehabilitation of the knee after surgery is directly connected to the functional outcome. Optimize the chances of a good functional outcome by being ready.

10) List what you are expecting to get out of surgery. Considering that severe pain and destruction of the knee joint is the main reason that knee arthroplasty is being scheduled, writing down what you would want to achieve will help you to fight for that

achievement after surgery, especially when physiotherapy is introduced during the rehabilitation period.

2) Knee replacement procedure

Step 1 - The surgeon makes an incision over the kneecap in a vertical direction to gain access to the knee joint. Incisions are often 4-10 inches in size, depending on the type of procedure. Smaller incisions are done for minimally invasive procedures.

Step 2 - The kneecap is removed from its position and diverted outside of the knee joint. This gives the surgeon access to the articulating surfaces of the bones that make up the knee.

Step 3 - The thighbone (femur) is the first bone to have its articular cartilage and defective surfaces cut off. After it is reshaped, the femoral artificial component is stuck in place by means of using bone cement.

Step 4 - The surgeon then removes the damaged tibial plateau surface, cutting off its entire cartilaginous surface. The bone is reshaped to match the shape of the artificial tibial component. The tibial component is unique in its structure. It is made up of 2 parts: the base and an insert. The metal base is initially glued in place by bone cement, and then a flexible plastic part is placed inside it. The second part of the tibial component acts as a shock absorber, and allows flexibility during knee joint flexion.

Step 5 - The patella is returned back in its place. However, its articular surface is also cut and replaced with an artificial component.

Step 6 - The now complete joint replacement is tested by the surgeon for stability and component adequacy. If the surgeon is satisfied by the construct, a drain is put into the knee for drainage, and the wound is closed. Wound closure can be by stitches or staples. Dressings are applied and the patient is taken to the recovery room.

3) Risks that come with knee arthroplasty

Like any other surgical intervention, knee replacement has some risks. These include:

-      Infection

-      Haematoma development

-      Iatrogenic neurovascular injury

-      Thromboembolism

-      Complications of anesthesia, where cardiac arrest is mentioned.

-      Failure

4) Post-operative adaptation

Analgesics are prescribed soon after surgery, usually narcotic types, to help ease the pain. Also, anticoagulants like heparin are given to prevent the development of thromboembolism, which is a possible complication in any major surgery. Its developmental risk is also increased if the patient is obese. The draining tube, which was left after surgery, is usually removed after 48-72 hours. Wound dressing after surgery is first done on the second day, after which the daily wound dressing is carried out.

Early immobilization is important for joint recovery. One thing for sure is that you will be able to do knee functions that you had refrained from doing before surgery, due to pain. Most patients stay in hospital for 3-7 days, then they are discharged.

5) After discharge

When you get home, help is usually required. If you follow the pre-op preparations discussed in this book, then you will be ready for recovery. Home arrangements should be done to ensure your safety in the house. For instance, slippery rugs should be removed, liquid spills should be wiped off immediately, and enough room should be created for you to be able to move around with your crutches. Your home assistant can assist you with medication taking and daily wound dressing. One should maintain normal eating habits, though this is difficult in the days soon after surgery. A balanced diet is good for recovery.

6) Adapting to the new joint

Unfortunately, adaptation is something that one has to learn by oneself, with time. Allow yourself to learn about the new joint quickly, yet cautiously.

- One has to get used to the clicks that occur during knee movement. This is normal and should not worry you. However, if any concerns are bugging you, always consult your doctor.

- Many patients often report itching around the incision site, and for some, small bumps even appear. Paraesthesia and leg numbness may also occur.

- There might be swelling soon after surgery. However, fever, chills, tenderness and pain in the knee are signs of an infection and one has to consult with their doctor if these arise. The incision site may also produce some watery discharge during an early infection. If the joint has been compromised by infection, the implant is usually taken out, and antibiotics are initiated to eradicate the infection.

- Avoid weight gain after a knee replacement. One has to remember that a surgeon chooses knee components using your age, weight and activity. Gaining weight will compromise the adequacy of the knee components.

- Weak legs are reported by most patients. This is mainly due to the fact that before surgery, most sufferers avoid activity because of pain, causing their muscles to weaken and atrophy. One target that a patient has to have post-surgery is to do knee strengthening exercises to improve leg strength and stability.

- A stiff knee is also common for a short period of time, but adequate physiotherapy during rehabilitation period will eliminate this complaint.

It is very important to note that artificial joints have a risk of failing with time, if they are subjected to heavy stress on a daily basis. Weight gain and high knee activity contribute to the chances of the constructs failing. This is why knee replacement in young adults is controversial. Read more on knee arthritis treatment by arthroplasty on Knee1.com, orthopaedics.about.com and orthoinfo.aaos.org.

7) How to be active with an arthroplasty

Most questions that come up are with reference to how one is to return to normal, daily activities. One has to gradually become active, while avoiding over stressing the joint. Your physical therapist should teach you some stretches and strengthening exercises that you can perform alone at home. The first 2-3 months post-surgery are critical for knee joint rehabilitation, and require a lot of effort from everyone involved, i.e. the patient and their physiotherapist.

Daily routine activities like driving are to be carefully introduced back into the schedule. Post-surgery, 3 months probation is often maintained, after which enough recovery is expected for you to be able to drive. Narcotic-based drugs and some other medications cause drowsiness, it is prohibited to drive if one is taking these medications. Sexual activity can be resumed in 6 weeks, and one has to be careful in knee positioning. Returning to work is usually possible at 2-3 months post-surgery; however, light duty is advised. Avoid carrying heavy things. Resuming sporting activity can be a big challenge, since someone may want to do a certain activity which is not permissible for people who have had knee arthroplasty. Golf, swimming, and cycling on a flat road are okay, while tennis, basketball, baseball and jogging are not good choices as they over stress the knee.

Chapter 5) How to eliminate arthritic knee pain

1) Knee arthritis diet

Dietary supplements are supportive additions to treatment of knee arthritis. This is true because a balanced diet is required for tissue repair after any form of injury. Bone and cartilage repair requires calcium, vitamin D, phosphorus and small quantities of other mineral elements. Your diet should include these nutrients to enhance recovery. Broccoli, beans, spinach, turnips, and nuts have calcium, while vegetable-based butters, mushrooms, and being in the sun for a few minutes during the day will help with sourcing vitamin D. Pumpkin and squash seeds, Brazil nuts, tofu and lentils are examples of phosphorus supplementary foods.

One doesn't necessarily have to be a vegan, but a vegetarian diet may help, since red meat has been associated with an increased risk of developing inflammatory arthritis. A vegetarian diet will also reduce saturated and poly-saturated fats in your diet, which will help in weight loss. So, diet maintenance will help in controlling body mass. One must try and control their body mass index by these dietary manipulations. Studies have shown that having too much adipose tissue in the body results in an enhanced inflammatory response, which is bad for arthritis. However, there are many types of knee arthritis, as we discussed, and each has its own developmental mechanism, so what is good for one individual may be symptom-aggravating in another. This is true because you will realize that sufferers tend to be picky about what they eat. And most nutritionists will tell you that in the foods that you are refraining from eating there are important nutrients that you should be getting in your diet. Selecting foods is thus controversial.

A knee arthritis diet should be rich in vitamins, antioxidants, minerals, essentials such as amino acids and fatty acids, and other nutrients. A healthy diet will strengthen your immunity and prevent simultaneous development of other medical conditions, e.g. pneumonia. Meat and saturated oils should be avoided; replacing them with fish oil or vegetable oils like olive oil may be beneficial. Plenty of fruits and vegetables are recommended; however, in a gouty knee, some vegetables like beans may worsen a flare-up. Also, cut down on sweet and sugary foods like cakes and biscuits. Deep-fried foods like samosas and fries are a no-no. Omega-3 is an essential fatty acid that is praised for its anti-inflammatory characteristics. Flax seeds, walnuts, sardines, soya beans and scallops are examples of foods that contain omega-3. In addition to relieving your joint pain, omega-3 also prevents depression, itchy skin, brittle nails and hair, and will improve your concentration. On the other hand, omega-6, which is found in butters, wheat germ, salad dressings and corn, may worsen inflammatory processes. It has been found to increase metabolic processes and may affect insulin production and enhance obesity. All these factors are not positive, as far as arthritis treatment is concerned. So, their use in the diet should be limited, and not completely excluded, since they also have some benefits to the body. Whenever fish oils are mentioned, it is important not to confuse with fish liver oils like cod liver oil. Fish liver oil is important in the diet as it helps in the absorption of Vitamin A. However, for arthritis treatment, it is fish oil that should be supplemented in large quantities. Taking a lot of fish liver oil will increase one's chance of suffering from Vitamin A overdose. So, just remember, the supplement that may be beneficial in knee arthritis is fish oil, and not fish liver oil.

Tips

➢ *Here are some recipes to try. They have been reported to be helpful by some sufferers; however, their research is very limited.*

➢ *To a cup of hot water, add 2 teaspoons of lemon juice and 1 teaspoon of honey, then drink twice daily.*

➢ *Drink alfalfa tea, twice daily.*

➢ *Rub warm vinegar on the painful joint before you go to bed.*

➢ *Try using shallaki, an Indian herb, which is applauded for its properties of improving blood flow to the knee joint. It's used especially in RA.*

➢ *Epsom salt baths are good for arthritis.*

➢ *Eating plenty of cherries is recommended to reduce any form of inflammation.*

2) Physiotherapy for knee arthritis

Physiotherapy is a branch of medicine that deals with the rehabilitation of individuals who suffer from movement disorders by means of exercise, equipment, education and motivation. Physiotherapists are professionals who perform physiotherapy, and like doctors, they are trained on the human body's anatomy, its physiology, how to diagnose diseases, and their treatments. Physiotherapists work hand in hand with rheumatologists, orthopedic surgeons, and sports medicine specialists because these professions complement each other.

The effectiveness of physiotherapy, in the treatment of knee arthritis, has been compared to knee arthroscopy. Some studies have shown that the outcome for patients who have had their OA treated by physiotherapy, and those who have had arthroscopic surgery, were similar. This does not only show the importance of physiotherapy in the treatment of arthritis, but also the unnecessary surgeries that are being performed in cases that would otherwise improve on conservative treatment.

When one selects a physiotherapist, remember that by law physiotherapists are required to be registered by the board of physiotherapy in your country. So, what you should be looking for is a board-certified, chartered physiotherapist.

Physiotherapists teach sufferers how to: improve knee joint mobility, strengthen knee muscles, and perform routine exercises.

Physiotherapy can help with pain management in arthritis treatment. This branch of medicine offers other measures for managing pain, e.g. ultrasound therapy, acupuncture, or shockwave therapy. These methods often require more than one session and as many as 3-4 sessions a week for several weeks to see the benefits.

a) Available physiotherapy pain management methods

- Traction

- Ultrasonic sound therapy

- Ice therapy

- Hot and cold therapy

- Electrical stimulation

- Heat therapy, e.g. wax bath

Posture also affects knee joint pain, and physiotherapists teach sufferers good posture and gait. Knee physio requires that one keeps active to keep up muscle strength and to keep the joint mobile.

The maintenance of joint function is offered by knee exercise. Controlled exercises help in strengthening knee muscles, ligaments and tendons, thus enhancing knee joint stability. Exercises performed in a swimming pool are great for starters; the buoyancy of your body in the water will assist movement. Hydrotherapy can effectively improve knee joint movement, muscle strength and general body fitness. Manual therapy is also helpful, especially in knees that have reduced mobility due to adhesions. Under anesthesia, physiotherapy passively stretches the joint to break free the adhesions. However, after any adhesion release, physiotherapy mobility exercises are aggressively implemented to prevent adhesions from reforming.

Physiotherapy also teaches patients how to use devices like splints, crutches, braces and walkers. Improper use of these items can cause further injury to the knee and/or cause a new condition altogether. Occupational therapy may also be introduced to knee arthritis treatment options to aid the overall functional outcome.

One should always start slowly, and gradually increase the intensity of the routines as the knee improves. Rest between activities is very crucial. However, if you have had a knee arthroplasty, consult your doctor on the type of movements that you should avoid to prevent joint dislocation. As much as exercise is necessary, you should avoid pushing the limit, as exercise can also worsen your arthritic knee. Rest during flare-ups, and commence with exercise when the inflammation has subsided.

b) Beneficial exercises for an arthritic knee

In physiotherapy, there are 3 types of exercises that are beneficial to knee arthritis treatment:

1) Stretches - to maintain function and mobility. These are often simple and specific.

2) Strengthening - these are muscle toning routines.

3) Supportive physio - e.g. aerobics, enhance the function of important body systems, i.e. circulatory and respiratory systems.

c) Benefits of physiotherapy in knee arthritis treatment

- Increases knee function

- Strengthens muscles, ligaments and tendons of the knee

- It's a healthy way of losing weight

- Reduces fatigue and depression

- Improves balance

- Improves posture and gait

- Improves sleeping patterns

- Contributes greatly to general body fitness

Tips

➢ *Check with your doctor before starting any new exercise routines.*

➢ *Make a timetable and calendar for your routine.*

➢ *Get motivation by inviting a friend or loved one to join in your exercise routine.*

➢   *List your main goals and the time duration that you expect to achieve those targets. Reward yourself on every achieved goal. Though one has to be realistic on the time estimates of attaining certain goals, physio takes some time for improvement to be evident, often 2-3 months.*

➢   *Review your achievements every 3 weeks, and modify the program if need be, e.g. to make it more interesting.*

d) Arthritic knee physio routines / exercises

Here are some exercises that you can try from home, though your doctor's advice is what matters the most.

It is very important that you get your doctor's advice prior to doing any of these exercises as I don't know your history of other medical issues you might suffer from.

A) Heel slides

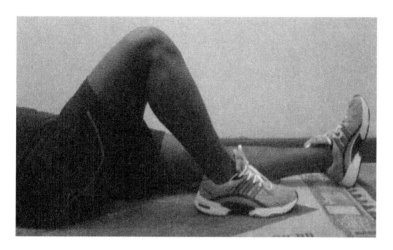

1) While lying on the bed/floor on your back, stretch both your legs straight in front of you, placing them together.

2) Keeping your heel on the bed/floor, slide your heel upwards as far as you can, bending your knee and hip in the process.

3) Hold the position for 4-6 seconds.

4) Slowly release to starting position.

5) Repeat the same procedure with your other leg.

6) Repeat 10-20 times, 3 times daily.

Tips

➢ *This exercise is good if done in the morning before getting out of bed. It loosens morning stiffness.*

➢ *Aim to bend the knee more every time.*

B) Long Arcs

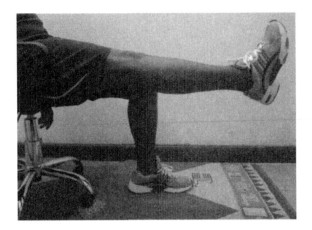

1) Sit on a chair with your back on the chair rest, and your knees bent, keeping them together.

2) Lift one leg up as much as you can, maintaining the knee in a straightened position.

4) Hold the position for 4-6 seconds.

5) Slowly lower your leg down to the floor, sliding your foot backwards under the chair, as far as you can.

6) Return to starting position, and do the same with the other leg.

7) Repeat for 10-20 times, 3 times daily.

Tips

➤ *This exercise is good if done every time you sit for more than 30 minutes. It helps in releasing knee stiffness.*

C) Quadriceps stretch

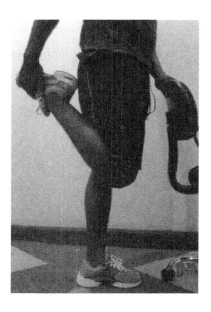

1) Stand straight behind a chair or table with your legs together.

2) Using the chair/table for balance, pull one heel towards your bottom, keeping your knees together and your back straight.

3) Pull the heel towards your bottom until you feel a stretch in front of your thigh.

4) Hold the position for 10 seconds and release.

5) Repeat 5 times, alternating the leg each time.

D) Hamstring stretch

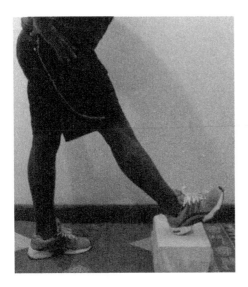

1) Stand straight behind a stair or step, with your legs together.

2) Put your hands on your hips, and place one heel of your foot on top of the stair or step, keeping your leg straight.

3) Lean your body forward at the hips, until you feel a stretch at the back of your thigh.

4) Hold the position for 10 seconds and release.

5) Repeat 5 times, alternating the leg each time.

E) Quads over fulcrum

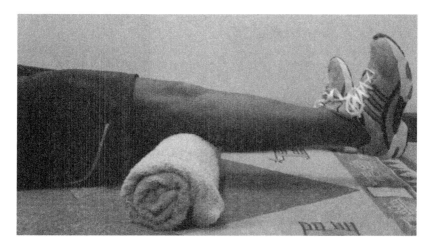

1) Lie straight on your back with a towel or foam roll under your knee.

2) Slowly raise your leg up, tightening the muscles in front of your thigh (Quadriceps muscle), though keeping the leg straight.

3) Hold the position for 4-6 seconds and release.

4) Repeat 8-10 times, 2 times daily.

F) Single leg stand

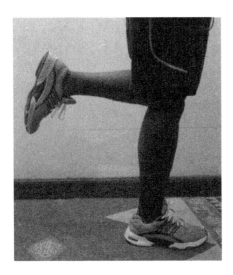

1) Stand straight with your feet together.

2) Lift your good leg up and stand on the arthritic leg for as long as you can manage.

3) Hold the position and release.

4) Repeat the process 5 times.

Tips

➢   *To enhance your balance, repeat the exercise with your eyes closed.*

➢   *Intensify the routine by throwing and catching a ball while you balance on the arthritic leg.*

G) Wall squats

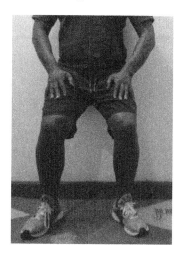

1) Stand with your feet apart and pointing forwards, at a distance of about 20 cm from a wall.

2) Place your back against the wall, maintaining the position of your feet.

3) Slowly slide down the wall as far as you can go, bending your knees as you do so.

4) Hold the position for 4-6 seconds and return to the starting position.

5) Repeat for 10-15 times, 3 times daily.

Tips

➢ *One can intensify this exercise by holding the position for more than 6 seconds.*

➢ *Sliding down deeper will also intensify the routine.*

H) Step ups

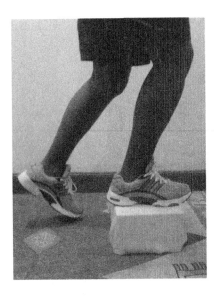

1) Stand in front of a step or stair.

2) Step up onto the step/stair using the arthritic leg first, followed by the normal leg.

3) Then step down using the normal leg first, followed by the arthritic leg.

4) Repeat this up-down stepping for 20-30 times.

Tips

➤　　　*This exercise is good for arthritic patients who have a staircase in their house.*

I) Sit to stand

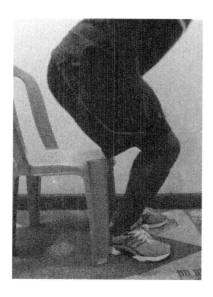

1) Place a chair in the middle of a room and sit on it.

2) Without holding anything for support, slowly stand up and sit back down.

3) Repeat this sitting and standing for 15-20 times.

Tips

➢   *This exercise is to be done slowly.*

➢   *Repeat the sit/stands many times for an intense routine.*

J) Leg stretch

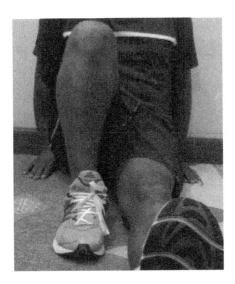

1) Sit on the floor with your back leaning on a wall.

2) Keep both your legs straight in front of you.

3) Slowly slide one leg up towards you as far as you can reach, bending your knee and keeping your foot flat on the ground.

4) Hold the position for 4-6 seconds.

5) Release and repeat the same with the other leg.

6) Repeat 8-10 times with each leg.

K) Knee dips

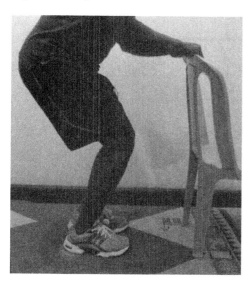

1) Stand straight behind a chair, with your legs together.

2) Holding the chair for support, bend your knees to a squatting position, as far down as you can go, maintaining a straight back.

3) Hold the squat for 10 seconds and release.

4) Repeat the knee dip 10-15 times, 2 times daily.

Tips

➢ *The deeper you go, the more intense the exercise.*

➢ *The longer you hold the dip, the more the routine is intensified.*

L) Leg criss-cross

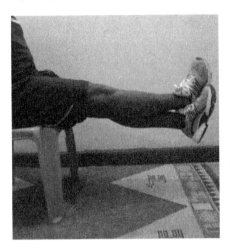

1) Sit on the edge of the bed or chair, with your legs crossed over each other, above the ground, in a straight position.

2) Push the leg on top downwards and the one below upwards.

3) Hold this position for 10 seconds, and feel your muscles stretch on your thighs.

4) Release and switch the leg position.

5) Repeat the routine 5 times on each leg.

Tips

➤ *This exercise is good if you do it in the morning as you get out of bed.*

M) Heel raise

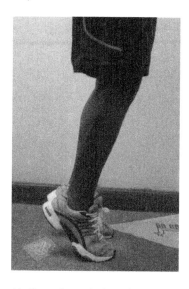

1) Stand straight with your feet together.

2) Raise both your heels up so that you stand on tiptoe.

3) Hold the position for 10 seconds.

4) Release and repeat 10 times.

Tips

➢   *Hold on to a chair or wall for support while you do this exercise.*

N) Hamstring bed sheet stretch

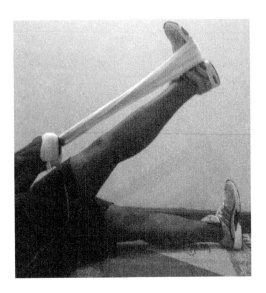

1) Lie down on your back with your legs stretched in front of you.

2) Loop a bed sheet around the middle of your foot.

3) Slowly pull on the bed sheet to pull the leg up in a straight position.

4) Hold for 15 seconds, and slowly bring it back down to the floor.

5) Switch the leg and repeat the routine.

6) Repeat the exercise 5-10 times on each leg.

O) Pillow squeeze

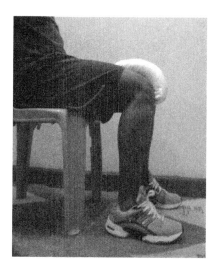

1) Sit on a chair with your knees bent together, and your feet flat on the ground.

2) Place a pillow between your knees.

3) Squeeze your knees together to squash the pillow.

4) Hold the position for 10 seconds.

5) Release and repeat 10 times.

P) Forward bend

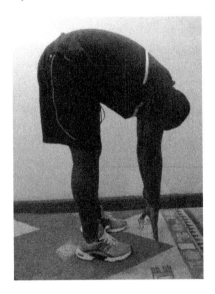

1) Stand straight with your legs together.

2) Bend your back forward to allow your fingers to touch your toes, keeping your legs and arms straight.

3) Hold the position for 5-10 seconds.

4) Slowly straighten your back up, and rest for 3 seconds.

5) Repeat the forward bend 10 times.

Tips

➢ *Individuals who suffer from knee arthritis also suffer from hip pain and lower back pain; this stretch will help relieve pain in these areas.*

Q) Resistance band hamstring curls

1) Tie a resistance band to the affected leg, with one end around your ankle, and the other around a table leg.

2) Lie straight on your abdomen in front of the table, folding your arms to support your head.

3) Slowly bend (flex) your knee while pulling the band, tightening the muscles in the back of your thigh (hamstrings).

4) Repeat curl 10 times.

Tips

➢   *Perform exercises when your knee is pain-free.*

➢   *Repeat exercise on the normal leg to equalize muscle loading.*

➢   *Repeat the curl more than 10 times for an intense workout.*

R) Resistance band extension stretch

1) Tie a resistance band on your affected leg, one end on your ankle, and the other on the leg of a chair.

2) Sit straight on the chair with your knees bent together.

3) Slowly straighten your knee, stretching the band as you do so.

4) Feel a stretch on your quadriceps muscle.

5) Release slowly to starting position.

6) Repeat the exercise 10 times and switch legs.

Tips

➢ *The tougher the band, the more intense the routine.*

➢ *The shorter the band, the better.*

S) The march

1) Sit straight on a chair with your knees bent together.

2) Move your knees up and down to perform a march, keeping your feet flat on the ground.

3) Repeat the march 20-30 times.

4) Rest for 1 minute and repeat the march once more.

Tips

➢ *This exercise is good when you have to sit for more than 20 minutes. It helps prevent a stiff knee.*

T) Knee raise

1) Lie straight on your back, with your arms on the side and feet together.

2) Press on your arms to support your body as you raise your buttocks off the ground.

3) Keep your feet flat on the floor.

4) Stretch your hips/pelvis up as far as you can go and hold the position for 5-10 seconds.

5) Release the hold and repeat routine 8-10 times.

U) Side slides

1) Lie straight on your back with your legs together.

2) Roll your legs outwards to point your foot to the side, though maintaining your kneecap in an upward position.

3) Hold for 4 seconds and roll your legs back in to starting position.

4) Repeat five times.

Tips

➢ *Useful as early rehab post knee arthroplasty*

V) Thigh squeeze

1) Lie flat on your back with your legs together.

2) Push the back of your knees down by tightening your thigh muscles.

3) Hold position for 6-8 seconds.

4) Release and repeat hold 3 times.

Tips

➤ *This exercise strengthens your quadriceps muscle, which is useful during walking and standing.*

➤ *This exercise is good during early rehab, post-knee arthroplasty.*

W) Passive hamstring stretch

1) Lie straight on your back with your legs together.

2) On the leg that had knee surgery, place a stack of pillows under your heel.

3) Hold the position for 10-15 minutes.

4) This will allow your new artificial knee to hang freely, thus stretching the joint.

Tips

➤ *This exercise is good for early rehab, post-arthroplasty of the knee. It allows full knee extension, which is important for walking.*

X) Straight leg lifts

1) Lie straight on your back, with your arms by your side and legs together.

2) Raise your operated leg straight up to about 6 inches off the ground.

3) Hold the position for 8-10 seconds.

4) Release and repeat 5 times.

Y) Ankle pumps

1) Lie straight on your back, with your arms by your side and legs together.

2) Move your toes on both feet up towards you, bending your ankle as far as you can go.

3) Hold for 6-8 seconds.

4) Release your hold and point your toes away from you, as far as you can go.

5) Hold the position for another 6-8 seconds.

6) Repeat routine 3 times on each side.

Z) Ankle rotations

1) Lie on a bed on your back, placing your feet straight on the edge of the bed.

2) Rotate 1 ankle in a clockwise direction 10 times, then anti clockwise.

3) Repeat the same with your other foot.

Tips

➢   *This exercise helps blood to flow back to your heart from your legs, hence is a great help in reducing swelling post-surgery.*

These are but a few available knee exercises. Your physiotherapist can teach you more routines, which are tailored to your specific individual requirements. Almost all exercise routines can be intensified by the use of weights and/or resistance bands. For instance, exercise G, the Wall squat, can be intensified by placing a Swiss ball behind you and conducting the exercise as described in this book. Swiss balls can be bought from any sports shop, or online. However, before intensifying any routine, consult your physiotherapist, whether or not your knees are ready for such intense stress application. Keeping your knees moving is a great way of maintaining function in knee arthritis.

For a total knee replacement, early rehab is crucial to attain initial range of motion, which is important for a successful recovery. Walking in the corridor for 3-5 minutes is good, several times a day. Then extend the walks as you gain confidence in your new artificial knee.

3) Home remedies for knee arthritis

Home remedies are additional things that a knee arthritis sufferer can try at home to make oneself more comfortable. However, it is important to keep in mind that these remedies will not provide some magical cure, but are a means to reduce the symptoms.

a) Drinks

Have fun trying some of these beverages.

1) Add half a teaspoon of devil's claw root to a cup of boiling water. Drink 1 cup daily.

2) Add 1 teaspoon of apple cider vinegar to a cup of warm water, then add a teaspoon of honey. Drink in the morning on alternate days.

3) Add a pinch of cinnamon powder to a cup of warm water, and then add a tablespoon of honey. Drink in the morning before having any breakfast, twice a week.

b) Teas

1) Green tea is good for weight loss.

2) White tea boosts the immune system and helps fight off infections.

3) Chamomile tea helps in wound healing and improves sleep patterns.

c) Herbs

1) Ginseng is a natural energy booster.

2) St. John's wort improves mood and prevents depression.

3) Boswellia, capsicum and licorice are good for knee pain relief.

d) Freestyle ideas

1) Eucalyptus oil - a small amount of eucalyptus oil is heated up and applied to the painful knee before bed.

2) Mustard plaster - add 1 part mustard powder to 1 part whole wheat flour, mix with enough water to form a paste. Apply this paste onto a cloth, and apply the cloth on the painful knee for 5-6 hours.

3) Apply a scarf over the knee or wear long johns when you stay up late to watch television. A shawl or small blanket covering the knees can suffice too.

4) Use celery in your daily recipes. Celery contains potassium, which has also been linked to knee joint pain if its intake is inadequate.

5) Keep well-hydrated.

6) For a gouty knee, avoid icing, as heat or cold therapies have been shown to be a waste of time in gout. Besides, it may add to your knee discomfort.

7) Eating a lot of apples is recommended for a gouty knee. Apples are said to neutralize uric acid.

8) Relax with burning lavender oil or lavender scented candles. This helps you sleep and it relieves stress.

9) For knee rheumatoid arthritis, which also affects the joints of the hands, one could use automatic appliances to do work, e.g. an electric can opener. Wearing electric gloves will also help to warm your hands and relieve tissue tension. Clever behavioral changes also help, e.g. using the elbow to open the door instead of a painful hand. Buy clothes with a zipper instead of buttons.

10) Ask for help to carry any heavy items.

11) Cherry juice, cherry compote, and cherry anything works.

4) Arthritic knee braces

Woman wearing a knee brace:

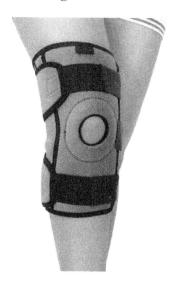

Arthritic knee braces are worn to offload some weight from the painful knee. They are chosen depending on the main effect desired. The level of support, specificity to disease condition, price, and brace style are some of the properties that are evaluated when choosing an arthritic knee brace. Knee braces aid in balance, therefore they prevent injuries such as falls. Pain relief has been reported by most brace users; however, more research is required on the functional outcomes of brace use.

It must be understood that arthritic knee braces do not cure arthritis, but they do help in alleviating knee joint pain. If one has never used any type of brace before, they may be uncomfortable in the early days of use. Knee braces are not substitutes to treatment; they are supportive measures to pain management. Consult your physiotherapist for helpful advice on how to choose a brace on an individual basis.

Types of arthritic knee braces

There are 3 main types of arthritic knee braces: sleeve, advanced knee brace, and unloading brace.

1) A sleeve is often made from neoprene. Their functions are mainly to provide compression and warmth. Sleeves can be hinged or non-hinged. A hinged knee brace would be the best choice for someone with side-to-side instability. The DonJoy Drytex hinged brace is a good example. Some exhibit a hole in front, which is there for extra comfort, since the hole helps to relieve pressure on the knee. Examples of general knee sleeves/supports are ACE brace with side stabilizers, and the Mueller wrap.

2) Advanced knee braces aid in supporting the knee joint and also reduce the weight that is applied on the knee joint. These kinds are used for moderate to severe knee arthritis, e.g. Neo G stabilized open support, McDavid pro-stabilizer and Mueller Hg80 knee brace. Some braces specifically seek to reduce pain; these include the DonJoy comfort knee brace and the Bort GenuZip knee brace.

3) Unloading knee braces are often used in knee OA, where compression to a reduced joint space helps reduce pain. The brace unloads weight off the region of severe pain by somewhat raising a compressed joint space, e.g. DonJoy OA Assist and DonJoy OA every day. One downside to this kind is that they are expensive, generally priced at $500 and more.

Arthritic knee braces can be bought online from: JointHealing.Com, breg.com, braceshop.com or PhysioRoom.com.

5) Maintaining activity with knee arthritis

Remaining active with knee arthritis is one of the challenges faced by most sufferers. Having to deal with things at a slower pace than usual can be frustrating. Accepting the reality of an arthritic knee is the greatest hurdle that one has to jump. Agreeing to not having the ability to perform your favorite hobby or activity is sad, but when things are beyond your control, you just have to deal with what you can control.

To stay active with an arthritic knee, it's just a matter of finding the best way of performing a particular activity. For those individuals who enjoy walks, using a cane for support will relieve pain from your knee, and it's a great way of maintaining your walking activity. One may also use the swimming pool to assist in walking. Walking in the shallow end is good, as the buoyancy of your body in the water will make your body light enough for your knees to function without any pain. For those who can swim, whilst you are still in the swimming pool, a few laps are a good way to stay generally fit, as swimming is one exercise that challenges all body muscles.

The type of shoes worn during an activity determines the comfort that one feels during their performance. High-heeled shoes increase the chances of arthritis and bunion development. Elevating the foot a few inches misaligns the body's weight-bearing angle; this is why high-heeled shoes are known for causing low back pain, foot arthritis and knee pain. The higher the shoe, the greater the risks. Flip-flops are yet another risk to your arthritic knee. They increase the risk of tripping and injuring oneself. A shoe with a soft, well-padded heel is great for walking, as it absorbs shock on uneven ground. Silicon insoles may also be used inside your shoes for enhanced comfort - they can be bought from Amazon.

A sufferer of knee arthritis should at all times maintain activity. It gives you a sense of well-being. The Center of Disease Control and Prevention (CDC) encourages arthritic patients to maintain activity and to refrain from the common mentality of wanting to completely rest your joints. In the Physical Activity Guidelines for Americans, people who suffer from arthritis are advised to follow either the active adult guideline or the active older adult guideline. Read more on physical activity and arthritis at cdc.gov.

SMART activity is what one should be aiming for. SMART is expanded as: S - start slow; M - modify your activity; A - activities should not cause you pain; R - recognizing safe activities for your knee; and T - talking to your doctor. Consult your doctor and come up with short-term and long-term methods of pain relief that you can use to ease pain. If pain is properly controlled, one is more likely to maintain activity. One may take pain medication such as ibuprofen before being active, though caution should be observed not to overdo the activity, since pain medication can mask injury. Losing weight will increase your performance during activity, as the body will not be fighting with other stresses. Excess weight puts more strain onto your knees.

Motivation during activity is also encouraging. Invite a friend to join in on the activity, or join community arthritis groups. If in your community there isn't a specific group for your needs, survey around if any exist elsewhere, or if it's possible to have one started in your area.

Making the activity fun will ensure that you remain active. For instance, fun video games which allow you to be off the couch like Wii Sports tennis by Nintendo are excellent substitutes to the usual outdoor activity. Planning home activities is another option. These activities include walking the dog, playing with your children or grandchildren, washing the car, gardening, and dancing through chores. Activities that involve a lot of squatting should be avoided.

Modifying daily chores can also be a great way of remaining active, e.g. parking in the last spot at a parking lot when you go shopping will increase the distance that you have to walk to and from the shop. For car drivers, instead of switching gears on manual transmission, automatic transmission may be an interesting modification.

After modifying daily chores to allow for free knee mobility, one might still use gadgets to aid this mobility. Knee braces, for example, can support your knee, securing it from buckling in or out when you walk. The different kinds of knee braces permit a choice of how your knee can be flexible with a brace. For instance, a hinged knee brace will still allow one to perform daily physio stretches while wearing it.

When the worst comes to worst, and one is completely disabled at the knees to move, electric mobility cars are a great advantage. They allow one to be independent in their own capacity. However, exercise of the other joints that are still mobile is a must to prevent their stiffness and a worsening disability category.

Summary

Knee arthritis is a medical condition that is affecting millions of people worldwide. It is an incurable disease, which, however, can be controlled by many efforts. Knee arthritis exists of many kinds, depending on the pathophysiological development of the disease. RA, gout, OA, SA, and post-traumatic arthritis are the frequently met arthritis types of the knee, hence they are the ones discussed in detail in this book. However, there are more than 100 recorded types of arthritis.

The predomination of knee arthritis is not in men or women, but depends on the specific type of knee arthritis. For instance, gout arthritis affects mostly men, while RA is more dominant in women. These are all epidemiological estimations of who gets affected by what; otherwise, knee arthritis can affect any individual at any age. Age groups in which knee arthritis develops also differ from one type of arthritis to another. An example being RA, it affects age ranges between 40-60 years, while post-traumatic arthritis affects any age, 5-10 years post knee injury.

One thing that is sure is that even though knee arthritis can affect anyone at any age, some individuals are susceptible to its development. Risk factors predispose people to the occurrence of knee arthritis. These risk factors generally include obesity, trauma, genetics, diet and some lifestyle choices such as smoking. Manipulating any one of the risk factors can be a preventative measure to the development of knee arthritis.

Knee arthritis is inflammation of the knee joint. This means that the components of the knee joint are injured in an arthritic knee. Injury is usually associated with erosion of the articular surfaces, synovial tissue hypertrophy with overproduction of synovial fluid, and the deformation of the knee joint structure. These changes lead to the knee joint being symptomatic.

Signs and symptoms of knee arthritis are often associated with pain, knee swelling, tenderness, warmth, and reduced knee mobility. Using the knee, in most cases, increases the intensity of pain. However, not all expected signs and symptoms should be present for a provisional diagnosis of knee arthritis to be made.

Knee arthritis diagnosis should be made by a doctor. This is of importance because any urgent diagnoses are excluded on time. A doctor diagnoses arthritis of the knee by means of: taking a complete medical history of an individual, a thorough general examination, and by additional medical tests. Blood works, which include FBC, CRP and ESR, are routine, while other specific blood tests such as rheumatoid factor and uric acid can also be ordered. Medical investigations that are usually ordered by doctors are X-rays, ultrasound, CT scan, and MRI. The main picture of an arthritic knee on X-ray is: reduced joint space, bony spurs, osteophytes, sclerotic bone margins, bone misalignments, i.e. genu valgus (knock-knees) or genu varus (bowlegs), and also marginal bone cysts. CT scans and MRI have a greater resolution power to X-rays, such that vascular injury or genesis, loose bodies in the knee joint, cartilage tears, meniscal tears, and ligament or tendon ruptures are clearly visualized. These additional medical tests aim to differentiate candidate diseases that might be applicable to a specific clinical picture presented by a sufferer.

After a knee arthritis diagnosis has been made, treatment is initiated. This treatment is initially aimed at reducing pain and inflammation. Medications such as NSAIDs, DMARDs and immunosuppressive medications are often used in treating knee arthritis. However, on their own these medications are inadequate. Supportive treatment plans including physiotherapy, diet, and education are a must. When all else fails, surgical treatment measures are sought. These include knee joint lavage, synovectomy, and arthroplasty.

The good news is that everyone will survive, since knee arthritis is not lethal.

I hope this book has been as informative as you expected it to be and more. For broadening your knowledge further on this subject, the following reads on Amazon may be of interest:

-       *Treat Your Own Knees; Simple Exercises to Build Strength, Responsiveness and Endurance,* by Jim Johnson

-       *Yoga for Arthritis: The Complete Guide,* by Loren Fishman and Ellen Saltonstall

- *The Fit Arthritic: Fighting Knee and Hip Arthritis with Exercise,* by Alan Kelton